INFLAMMATION THE SILENT FIRE: COMBAT CHRONIC INFLAMMATION WITH A SCIENCE-BASED APPROACH

PROVEN STRATEGIES TO RESTORE YOUR IMMUNE SYSTEM, REDUCE STRESS, AND IMPROVE GUT HEALTH TO START FEELING YOUR BEST

DR. CARLY STEWART - DPT

This book is dedicated to all those who struggle with chronic inflammation, who face each day not knowing if they will find relief from their pain. To the warriors who fight an invisible battle and strive tirelessly for a semblance of normalcy and well-being amidst the challenges.

To my patients, whose resilience and courage inspire me every day—this book is for you. Your stories and experiences have not only influenced these pages but have also deepened my understanding and compassion as a practitioner.

And to my family and friends, for your unwavering support and patience through the long hours and the endless pursuit of healing—this journey would not have been possible without you.

May this book light your path to recovery and guide you to a healthier, more vibrant existence, liberated from the constraints of inflammation.

PRAISE FOR
DR. CARLY STEWART - DPT

If you're searching for a clear, actionable plan to reduce inflammation and enhance your overall health, this book is an essential resource. Packed with evidence-based strategies, it demystifies the science of inflammation and provides practical advice that can dramatically improve your quality of life. Whether you are dealing with chronic inflammation or just interested in preventive health, these insights are invaluable. A must-read for anyone serious about reclaiming their health.

— DR. JAMES MACKAY, MD

As a podiatrist, dealing with inflammation, particularly patients with diabetes, is a daily challenge. This book provides straightforward, practical strategies to manage and reduce chronic inflammation naturally. Anyone looking to relieve pain and improve their health will find it invaluable. It's a guide worth having in your collection.

— HARMINDER RAYAT - B.HSCI. M. POD MAPODA

CONTENTS

FOREWORD

Foreword by Dr. James Mackay, MD

As a practicing physician who deals with inflammatory diseases, I have sought to understand and combat the conditions that stem from chronic inflammation. It's a pervasive problem—one that can significantly deteriorate quality of life —yet it's also one of the most manageable. It gives me great pleasure to introduce this essential guide aimed at demystifying chronic inflammation and providing readers with effective strategies to alleviate it.

Chronic inflammation is the body's persistent, harmful response to long-term irritants or injuries. It plays a central role in a host of common diseases, including but not limited to IBD, cardiovascular diseases, diabetes, arthritis, and various neurological conditions. The processes involved are complex and can lead to a vicious cycle of damage if not appropriately addressed.

This book lays out specific, scientifically supported steps to help reduce inflammation naturally. These strategies range from adopting anti-inflammatory diets and improving gut health to reducing stress, enhancing sleep quality, and incorporating regular physical activity.

Each recommendation is rooted in solid research and is explained here with clarity and precision.

What sets this book apart is its practical approach. The advice it offers goes beyond the theoretical, offering real, actionable steps that individuals can take to improve their health. It is written with the understanding that while the changes may be challenging, the rewards—reduced pain, increased energy, and overall better health—are well worth the effort.

Moreover, the book stresses that managing chronic inflammation is not about seeking quick fixes but about making sustainable lifestyle changes. This perspective is crucial because true health does not come from a pill or a temporary diet but from a consistent, thoughtful approach to living.

I recommend this book enthusiastically to anyone who suffers from chronic inflammation, or anyone who aims to improve their overall health through informed, practical changes in their lifestyle. Whether you are just starting to experience symptoms or have been managing inflammation for years, the strategies outlined here can significantly improve your quality of life.

To your health and well-being,

Dr. James Mackay, MD

Fellow of the Royal Australian College of General Practitioners

FREE ANTI-INFLAMMATORY DIET COOKBOOK

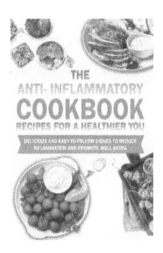

To show my gratitude for your purchase of Inflammation: The Silent Fire, I have included a complimentary anti-inflammatory diet cookbook to aid in your health journey.

Please follow the link or use the QR code to receive your free copy.

https://rehabmentor.ck.page/

INTRODUCTION

Think of this book as a call to action to slow down, breathe, and allow your body to do what it does best —heal.

- Will Cole

Have you ever wondered about the whispers of discomfort—those subtle signals that something might be amiss within? These whispers, often dismissed as mere nuisances, could be the voice of chronic inflammation—a silent fire smoldering within.

So, take a moment to pause and reflect. Perhaps it was the persistent bloating after meals, the inexplicable fatigue that weighed you down each morning, or the nagging joint pain that seemed to flare up at the most inconvenient times.

In these moments, it is easy to dismiss these whispers of discomfort as nothing more than the occasional inconvenience of modern life. Yet, what if these signals were trying to tell you something more profound? What if they were the body's way of signaling that something deeper and more insidious might be at play?

Chronic inflammation, often overlooked and underestimated, could be the silent culprit behind these seemingly unrelated symptoms. It is like a smoldering fire quietly burning beneath the surface—its presence masked by the hustle and bustle of daily life. But make no mistake; this silent fire can wreak havoc on our health and sow the seeds of disease and discomfort if left unchecked.

But here is the thing about chronic inflammation—it is not an inevitable part of aging, nor is it a fate we must resign ourselves to. Instead, it is a dynamic process—one that can be influenced and modulated by our lifestyle choices, habits, and even mindset. Our power lies in recognizing that we have the ability to shape our health with each choice.

Many of us know the feeling all too well—the persistent, unexplained discomfort that lingers in the background of our lives, clouding our days with fatigue, joint pains, and a sense of unease. We seek answers, desperate to understand why these symptoms persist and how they relate to our health's broader tapestry.

For some, it is the relentless onslaught of stress-related symptoms: headaches that refuse to abate, digestive issues that disrupt daily life, or insomnia that robs us of precious sleep. We are left grappling with the relentless demands of modern life, searching for insights into the tangled web of stress, cortisol levels, and chronic inflammation, and yearning for effective equilibrating strategies.

And then there are those who have traversed the winding paths of conventional medicine only to find themselves disillusioned with the results. Despite trying every pill, potion, and prescription in the book, their symptoms persist leaving them disheartened and disenchanted with the notion of a one-size-fits-all solution. They crave alternatives that offer a glimmer of hope in a sea of uncertainty.

But, perhaps amidst the chaos and confusion, there is a flicker of awareness—a recognition that our symptoms are not isolated islands but interconnected within our existence. We yearn for a holistic solution, one that embraces the totality of our being—mind, body, and spirit—and offers a comprehensive understanding of how lifestyle factors, diet, and other elements contribute to chronic inflammation.

In moments of vulnerability and uncertainty, this book provides science-backed strategies for healing and wholeness, giving us hope and empowering us to take charge of our well-being.

So, to those who find themselves wrestling with unexplained discomfort, navigating the turbulent waters of stress-related symptoms, or seeking solace in the midst of dissatisfaction with conventional approaches: Know that you are not alone. Together, we will traverse this terrain with compassion, curiosity, and courage while uncovering the secrets of chronic inflammation and unlocking the keys to vibrant health and vitality.

And why should you listen to me? Because I have walked the path you are on and have felt the ache of unexplained discomfort, the weight of stress-related symptoms, and the frustration of seeking answers using conventional approaches while grappling with the relentless grip of chronic inflammation, trying to make sense of it all.

For the past four years, I have been dealing with and managing severe ulcerative colitis—a journey that has taught me more about pain and inflammation than any textbook ever could. Through the highs and lows of my own inflammatory journey, I have gained a deep understanding of the struggles faced by those with autoimmune conditions and chronic inflammation.

With a background in physical therapy, I bring a unique blend of scientific expertise and practical knowledge to this book. Drawing from my experiences in understanding the intricacies of the human body and its response to various stimuli, I am well-positioned to offer valuable insights into the connections between chronic inflammation and physical well-being.

In addition to professional expertise, it is my passion for empowering individuals to take control of their health that drives me forward. I believe in the power of education, transformative potential of knowledge, and profound impact that small, intentional changes can have on our lives.

Through this book, I aim to bridge the gap between scientific knowledge and practical application offering you a holistic guide that encompasses not only the physiological aspects of inflammation but also actionable steps rooted in the principles of physiotherapy. This approach ensures that you—regardless of your background—can navigate the complexities of chronic inflammation with confidence and embark on a journey towards lasting health and vitality.

Imagine waking up each morning feeling refreshed and rejuvenated —your body humming with vitality and energy. Gone are the days of dragging yourself out of bed weighed down by the burden of chronic fatigue. Instead, you greet each day with a renewed sense of purpose and enthusiasm eager to embrace the opportunities that lie ahead.

As you go about your day, you move with ease and grace with supple joints free from the stiffness that once plagued you. The persistent ache in your back and nagging pain in your knees—they are nothing more than distant memories fading into oblivion as your body finds its natural rhythm once more.

At meal times, you savor the vibrant flavors of nutrient-rich foods knowing that each bite is nourishing your body from the inside out. Gone are the days of mindless eating and empty calories. Instead, you approach food with intention, fueling your body with the building blocks it needs to thrive.

But it is not just your physical health that undergoes a transformation—it is your mental and emotional well-being too. The cloud of stress that once hung heavy over your head dissipates replaced by a sense of calm and clarity. You no longer find yourself swept away by the relentless demands of life; rather, you meet each challenge with resilience and grace.

And as you reflect on your journey—the ups and downs, triumphs and setbacks—you realize that you have become the architect of your own health destiny. Armed with knowledge and empowered by experience, you have silenced the fire of chronic inflammation and ignited a spark of vitality that burns brightly within you.

This is the promise that awaits you on the other side of this journey —a future filled with health, vitality, and boundless potential. So, take my hand, and let us embark on this journey together. Together, we will silence the fire of chronic inflammation and unlock the door to a future of limitless possibilities.

CHAPTER I

UNDERSTANDING CHRONIC INFLAMMATION

"The research is clear: if you can keep your body relatively free of chronic inflammation, you will increase your likelihood of living a long and healthy life."

- Dr. Mehmet Oz

I magine chronic inflammation as a smoldering fire within the body, silently consuming its resources. Knowledge acts as the water needed to douse these flames, preventing the fire from spreading and causing further damage. It becomes a critical tool in our firefighting arsenal, enabling us to identify the sources of the blaze within our bodies, interpret the distress signals they emit, and commence the firefighting efforts needed for recovery. With every new insight into our health, we're effectively adding more water to our firefighting arsenal, gaining the power to extinguish the fire of inflammation before it becomes a wildfire.

In the context of chronic inflammation, understanding becomes not just a source of strength but a vital rescue line. It serves as the gateway to unraveling the complexities of our physiology, the tool for interpreting the messages our bodies relay, and the initial stride towards healing.

Navigating health-related discussions can sometimes feel like trying to find one's way through dense smoke, whether it's sitting in a healthcare provider's office, outwardly agreeing while internally lost in confusion, or searching the internet for answers, only to be overwhelmed by a cloud of medical jargon that obscures more than it clarifies. However, the truth shines through like a beam from a firefighter's flashlight: Medical conditions are not inescapable infernos but fires that can be controlled and extinguished with the right knowledge. This chapter is dedicated to offering you that crucial key, aimed at quenching the embers of chronic inflammation and arming you with the knowledge needed to navigate your way back to health.

THE DUAL NATURE OF INFLAMMATION

At its core, inflammation is not an enemy but a fire alarm within our body's complex ecosystem, a vital signal in our body's natural defense mechanism. Envision acute inflammation as the emergency response team's first line of defense, a rapid activation to combat the flames of injury, illness, or invasion. This inflammation is the body's initial spark, its way of calling in the fire brigade to defend against foreign invaders such as bacteria and viruses, a dedicated team fighting tirelessly against illness, and the medics on the ground, facilitating healing and recovery from the damage inflicted.

Inflammation is a natural physiological process that signals our body to pay attention and take action when something goes wrong. Imagine when you accidentally cut your finger while chopping vegetables or scrape your knee while falling off a bike. Your body immediately springs into action, initiating inflammation to help heal the wound. Special immune cells rush to the site of injury, releasing chemicals that increase blood flow and make the area swell, turn red, and feel warm. This is your body's way of sending reinforcements to fight off any germs and start repairing the damage. Similarly, when you catch a cold or get a fever, inflammation kicks in to help your body fight off the invading germs. It is a protective response designed to keep you healthy and safe.

So, inflammation is not always a bad thing—it is actually a vital part of your body's defense system, helping you heal and stay well.

DEFINING CHRONIC INFLAMMATION

Chronic inflammation is a superhighway that runs straight to the most deadly diseases out there...Chronic inflammation comes from how we think, how we feel, and how we live.

— Jeffrey Rediger

Sometimes, the inflammation process does not stop when it should. Even after the injury has healed or the infection has cleared, the alarm system in our bodies continues to blare incessantly in the background, even though there is no real danger. This is what we call chronic inflammation.

This persistent inflammation can wreak havoc on our bodies. Instead of protecting us, it starts to cause problems. Imagine if your house alarm went off constantly—day and night—without any real threat. Eventually, you would become exhausted, frazzled, and unable to relax or focus on anything else. Similarly, chronic inflammation can wear down our bodies leading to a host of health issues.

It is like a slow-burning fire smoldering beneath the surface and damaging our tissues and organs over time, often ignored or underestimated because its symptoms are neither immediate nor glaring. This ongoing inflammation has been linked to a range of health

3

problems including heart disease, diabetes, arthritis, and even cancer. So, while inflammation is a necessary part of our body's defense system, chronic inflammation can be harmful, and it is important to understand how to manage it effectively.

This persistent inflammation can be caused by lots of things like unhealthy eating habits, exposure to toxins, or even stress. It is like our bodies are constantly under attack, and our immune system is always on high alert, trying to put out the fire. We will talk more about the causes in Chapter 2.

DIFFERENTIATING FROM ACUTE INFLAMMATION

Acute inflammation is a physiological response characterized by the body's rapid reaction to harmful stimuli such as injury or infection. It serves as a protective, short-term mechanism aimed at eliminating the initial cause of cell injury, clearing out damaged tissue, and initiating the healing process. This response involves the recruitment of immune cells and the release of inflammatory mediators to the affected site, therefore, facilitating the removal of pathogens and restoration of tissue integrity.

In contrast, chronic inflammation signifies a state of inflammation that is both dysregulated and prolonged, persisting long after the resolution of the initial insult. Unlike acute inflammation, which is characterized by its transient and localized nature, chronic inflammation involves sustained activation of immune cells and continuous production of inflammatory mediators throughout the body.

This persistent inflammatory response can have detrimental effects leading to progressive tissue damage, compromised organ function, and the onset or exacerbation of a range of chronic diseases. The prolonged presence of inflammatory signals disrupts the delicate balance of the immune system, thus, resulting in a cascade of cellular and molecular events that contribute to chronic tissue injury and dysfunction.

Over time, this chronic inflammatory burden can inflict cumulative harm on various organ systems, ultimately culminating in the manifestation of chronic conditions such as cardiovascular disease, metabolic disorders, neurodegenerative diseases, and autoimmune disorders. Recognizing the insidious nature of chronic inflammation is imperative for implementing targeted interventions aimed at restoring immune homeostasis and mitigating the adverse consequences associated with persistent inflammatory activation.

FORMS OF CHRONIC INFLAMMATION

Chronic inflammation—like a persistent shadow looming over our bodies—manifests in various forms with their own distinct characteristics and consequences. From the silent infiltration of low-grade systemic inflammation to the localized battlegrounds of autoimmune disorders and the intricate interplay of metabolic disturbances and neuroinflammatory storms, the spectrum of chronic inflammation encompasses a myriad of complexities.

Understanding the diverse manifestations of chronic inflammation is paramount, as it empowers us to recognize the signs, intervene effectively, and embark on a journey towards restoration and vitality.

LOW-GRADE SYSTEMIC INFLAMMATION

Low-grade systemic inflammation is like a stealthy intruder affecting the whole body. Its constant presence quietly causes trouble in the background.

Eating too much unhealthy food, not getting enough exercise, or being exposed to toxins in the environment are all triggers. Our bodies are constantly being attacked, triggering a relentless assault on our immune system. It's as if our immune defenses are under a perpetual siege, always in a state of heightened alert, tirelessly trying to fend off these invisible threats.

Chronic inflammation is a pervasive and subtle condition that can have significant impact on our overall health. It is a slow-burning ember that lingers beneath the surface and can contribute to the development of various diseases over time.

For instance, it can lead to the build-up of plaque in our arteries, which is a precursor to heart conditions. Additionally, it can affect the body's ability to process sugar effectively, leading to insulin resistance and the onset of diabetes. Chronic inflammation has also been linked to mental health issues, such as depression. Therefore, it is clear that this low-grade inflammation can have a profound impact on both our minds and bodies.

LOCALIZED CHRONIC INFLAMMATION

Localized chronic inflammation is when inflammation affects specific parts of the body. Like a fire that is contained in just one room of a house, it still causes damage.

For example, arthritis is a type of localized inflammation that affects the joints causing pain, swelling, and stiffness. Inflammatory bowel disease (IBD) is another example, when intestinal inflammation leads to symptoms like abdominal pain and diarrhea. Chronic respiratory conditions like asthma and chronic bronchitis are also caused by localized inflammation in the lungs, subsequently causing difficult breathing (dyspnea).

AUTOIMMUNE INFLAMMATION

Autoimmune inflammation is the mistaken perception of the body's immune system of its own tissues as threats to be attacked. In autoimmune diseases like rheumatoid arthritis (RA), lupus, and psoriasis, the immune system goes haywire, thus, launching attacks on healthy tissues instead of germs or foreign invaders.

These conditions can cause a range of symptoms—from joint pain and swelling in RA to skin rashes and fatigue in lupus. The up close and personal battle of our bodies leads to chronic inflammation and ongoing health problems.

METABOLIC INFLAMMATION

Metabolic inflammation delves into the complex relationship between inflammation and metabolic disorders such as obesity and insulin resistance. Inflammation sets up camp in our bodies' metabolic pathways, hence, disrupting the delicate balance of energy regulation.

In conditions like obesity, inflammation can arise within adipose tissue—the fat cells in our bodies—due to factors like an unhealthy diet, a sedentary lifestyle, and genetic predisposition. This adipose tissue inflammation can spill over into the bloodstream, subsequently triggering systemic inflammation and contributing to metabolic dysfunction.

This systemic inflammation can interfere with insulin signaling leading to insulin resistance—a hallmark of type 2 diabetes mellitus (DM2). It creates a vicious cycle where inflammation and metabolic dysfunction feed off each other, hence, exacerbating health issues and increasing the risk of chronic diseases.

NEUROINFLAMMATION

Neuroinflammation shines a light on inflammation happening within the central nervous system—our body's command center. Neuroinflammation is a storm brewing in our brains causing disturbances in the delicate balance of neural function.

In neurodegenerative diseases like Alzheimer's and multiple sclerosis, neuroinflammation plays a key role in driving disease progression. It poses a relentless assault on the brain and spinal cord, therefore, leading to the destruction of nerve cells and the formation of scar tissue.

These conditions can cause a range of symptoms—from memory loss and cognitive decline in Alzheimer's to numbness and paralysis in multiple sclerosis.

INFLAMMATORY RESPONSES IN AGING

Inflammatory responses in aging shed light on the intricate relationship between inflammation and the natural aging process. It is like a slow burn that gradually intensifies as we grow older, consequently impacting various aspects of our health and well-being.

Chronic inflammation may contribute to age-related diseases and physiological decline by promoting tissue damage, impairing cellular function, and disrupting metabolic homeostasis.

As we age, our bodies become more susceptible to chronic inflammation leading to an increased risk of conditions like cardiovascular disease, osteoarthritis, and cognitive decline. As a ticking time bomb hidden in the background, chronic inflammation waits to unleash its destructive potential.

BIOLOGICAL MECHANISMS BEHIND CHRONIC INFLAMMATION

Chronic inflammation is underpinned by complex biological processes primarily driven by dysregulated immune responses. Immune cells—crucial components of the body's defense system—play pivotal roles in recognizing and eliminating foreign invaders and damaged cells. However, in chronic inflammatory conditions, this immune surveillance system malfunctions, thus leading to sustained and excessive inflammation (Pahwa & Jialal, 2019).

The activation of immune cells—characterized by a persistent release of inflammatory mediators—is central to chronic inflammation. This dysregulation may arise from genetic predispositions, environmental factors, and lifestyle choices. Genetic variations can predispose individuals to heightened immune reactivity, while environmental triggers such as pollutants and infections can exacerbate inflammatory responses. Additionally, lifestyle factors including an unhealthy diet, sedentary behavior, chronic stress, and poor sleep hygiene can further fuel immune dysregulation.

Understanding the interplay between immune cells and chronic inflammation is essential for developing targeted interventions to mitigate its effects. By elucidating the underlying mechanisms driving immune dysfunction, individuals can adopt proactive strategies to modulate their immune responses, address contributing factors, and alleviate the burden of chronic inflammation on their health and well-being.

CYTOKINES AND MOLECULAR PROCESSES

Within the realm of chronic inflammation, cytokines play pivotal roles in regulating inflammatory responses. These small proteins act as messengers facilitating communication between immune cells and coordinating the body's defense mechanisms. In chronic inflammatory states, the production of cytokines becomes dysregulated resulting in an imbalance between pro- and anti-inflammatory signals.

Pro-inflammatory cytokines, such as tumor necrosis factor-alpha (TNF-α), interleukin-1 (IL-1), and IL-6, promote inflammation by activating immune cells and stimulating the production of inflammatory mediators. Conversely, anti-inflammatory cytokines, such as IL-10 and transforming growth factor beta (TGF-β), counteract inflammation by inhibiting immune responses and promoting tissue repair (Saini et al., 2005).

The molecular processes underlying chronic inflammation involve a complex interplay of signaling pathways and cellular interactions. Persistent activation of immune cells, specifically macrophages and T cells, leads to sustained cytokine production and inflammatory mediator release. These inflammatory mediators, including prostaglandins, leukotrienes, and reactive oxygen species (ROS), further amplify the inflammatory response and contribute to tissue damage and dysfunction (Chen et al., 2017).

Understanding the role of cytokines and molecular processes in chronic inflammation provides valuable insights into the mechanisms driving inflammatory diseases. By targeting specific cytokines or signaling pathways, researchers and clinicians can develop novel therapeutic approaches aimed at modulating immune responses and restoring immune homeostasis. Additionally, elucidating the molecular underpinnings of chronic inflammation may pave the way for the identification of biomarkers for early disease detection and monitoring, ultimately improving patient outcomes and quality of life (QOL).

I understand that the concepts of cytokines and molecular processes may seem complex and challenging to grasp at first glance, but rest assured, you do not need to be a scientist to understand their significance. What truly matters is recognizing the impact they have on our health and well-being.

IMPLEMENTING INSIGHTS

- Chronic inflammation is a prolonged and dysregulated immune response that can contribute to the development of various health issues.
- Identifying the differences between acute and chronic inflammation is crucial for understanding their respective impacts on the body.

- By understanding the biological mechanisms driving chronic inflammation, you can take proactive steps to manage and mitigate its effects on their health and well-being.

ACTIONABLE CHECKLIST

- Take time to learn about chronic inflammation and its implications for overall health.
- Reflect on your personal health history and identify potential signs or symptoms of chronic inflammation.
- Consider consulting with a healthcare professional for further evaluation and guidance.
- Begin incorporating anti-inflammatory lifestyle changes such as adopting a balanced diet, engaging in regular physical activity, and managing stress effectively.

Continuing our journey into the realm of chronic inflammation, we now delve into Chapter 2, where we uncover the concealed risks associated with persistent inflammation and explore how it impacts our health and QOL.

CHAPTER 2
THE HIDDEN DANGERS OF CHRONIC INFLAMMATION

There is overwhelming evidence for a strong association between inflammation and depression.

- Edward Bullmore

Let me share a personal journey that sheds light on the profound impact of this silent assailant. My own struggles with chronic inflammation not only challenged my physical well-being but also profoundly influenced every aspect of my life. From the relentless fatigue that clouded my days to the persistent discomfort that haunted my nights, the insidious nature of chronic inflammation cast a shadow over my existence quietly eroding my vitality and diminishing my QOL. Yet, through these trials, I gained invaluable insights into the hidden dangers lurking beneath the surface, which drove me to unravel the mysteries of chronic inflammation and its far-reaching consequences.

ROLE IN VARIOUS DISEASES AND HEALTH CONDITIONS

As initially mentioned in Chapter 1, chronic inflammation plays an immense role in several diseases and health conditions.

HEART DISEASE

Chronic inflammation can have a significant impact on heart health, as it contributes to the development and progression of various cardiovascular conditions. One of the key ways in which chronic inflammation affects the heart is through a process called atherosclerosis.

Chronic inflammation plays a critical role in the development of atherosclerosis by triggering an inflammatory response within the arterial walls (Rafieian-Kopaei et al., 2014). As a response to the chronic inflammation, as in other instances and tissues, macrophages activate and subsequently accumulate in the arterial walls. The inflamed, thus, damaged arteries are vulnerable to buildup of plaque in the arteries made up of fatty deposits, cholesterol, calcium, and other substances found in the blood.

Progressive plaque growth and hardening narrows the arteries and restricts blood flow to the heart. This reduced blood flow can deprive the heart muscle of oxygen and nutrients, thus, increasing the risk of serious cardiovascular events such as heart attacks and strokes.

Furthermore, chronic inflammation can also contribute to other cardiovascular issues such as hypertension (high blood pressure) and arrhythmias (irregular heart rhythms). Inflammation can disrupt the normal functioning of blood vessels and the heart, consequently leading to elevated blood pressure and disturbances in heart rhythm.

DIABETES

Chronic inflammation can have a profound impact on insulin resistance and diabetes onset. Insulin resistance occurs when the body's cells become less responsive to insulin—a hormone produced by the pancreas that helps regulate blood sugar levels.

When chronic inflammation is present in the body, it can disrupt the normal functioning of insulin and interfere with its ability to effectively regulate blood sugar levels. This can lead to insulin resistance where the cells become less responsive to insulin's signals, resulting in elevated blood sugar levels.

Furthermore, chronic inflammation can also contribute to the progression of diabetes by damaging the insulin-producing cells in the pancreas. Over time, this damage can impair the pancreas's ability to produce insulin, hence, further exacerbate insulin resistance and lead to elevated blood sugar levels.

In addition to promoting insulin resistance and impairing insulin production, chronic inflammation can also contribute to the development of complications associated with diabetes. These complications include cardiovascular disease, kidney disease, nerve damage, and vision problems.

ARTHRITIS AND AUTOIMMUNE DISORDERS

Arthritis refers to a group of conditions characterized by inflammation of the joints leading to pain, stiffness, and swelling. Chronic inflammation plays a central role in the development and progression of arthritis by damaging the joints and surrounding tissues (Senthelal & Thomas, 2018).

When articular chronic inflammation occurs, it can trigger an immune response that leads to the destruction of cartilage and bone. This inflammatory process can result in the characteristic symptoms of arthritis such as joint pain, stiffness, and decreased range of motion.

In addition to arthritis, chronic inflammation can also contribute to the development of autoimmune disorders. Chronic inflammation plays a critical role in the pathogenesis of autoimmune disorders by driving the immune system's aberrant response.

In autoimmune disorders, chronic inflammation can cause the immune system to produce antibodies that target healthy tissues leading to inflammation and damage. This immune-mediated inflammation can affect various organs and tissues in the body resulting in a wide range of symptoms and complications.

LONG-TERM EFFECTS ON QUALITY OF LIFE

Indeed, the diseases instigated by inflammation have a considerable impact on one's QOL, often triggering additional health complications that compound the challenges faced. Chronic inflammation presents formidable barriers to completing mundane tasks and leaves individuals grappling with persistent fatigue and malaise.

The physical manifestations of inflammation such as pain, stiffness, and discomfort pervade the body, thereby impeding mobility and curtailing the pursuit of pleasurable activities. For instance, individuals grappling with arthritis find themselves confronted with inflamed joints that hinder basic movements like walking, ascending stairs, or even grasping objects. Such limitations extend beyond mere physical impediments permeating various facets of daily existence. The ability to fulfill occupational duties, attend to personal care needs, and partake in meaningful interactions with loved ones becomes compromised, therefore, amplifying feelings of frustration and isolation.

Furthermore, the pervasive nature of chronic inflammation extends its reach beyond physical discomfort; seeping into the realms of energy and mood regulation, it takes a multifaceted toll on one's well-being. Persistent inflammation often saps away vitality and exacerbates emotional distress, thereby leaving individuals grappling with profound fatigue and irritability.

Chronic inflammation can also disrupt our sleep patterns by creating a vicious cycle that worsens inflammation and impacts our overall well-being. High inflammation levels can interfere with our body's ability to regulate sleep hormones like melatonin making it difficult to fall or stay asleep throughout the night. As a result, we may find ourselves tossing and turning, waking up frequently, or struggling to achieve deep, restorative sleep.

Sleep deprivation triggers the release of stress hormones like cortisol, which in turn promotes inflammation. This sets off a harmful cycle where inflammation disrupts sleep, hence, positively reinforcing itself and ultimately leading to a decline in our physical and mental health.

The consequences of disrupted sleep can ripple throughout our lives affecting our mood, cognitive function, immune system, and overall ability to function optimally. Therefore, addressing sleep problems is crucial to managing chronic inflammation and promoting better health outcomes.

The disruptive influence of inflammation is not confined to the waking hours alone; it infiltrates the realm of slumber, therefore, sabotaging the restorative process of sleep and depriving individuals of the rejuvenation essential for daily functioning. This perpetual cycle of discomfort and exhaustion forms an insidious barrier to cultivating a fulfilling existence, impedes the pursuit of once-cherished activities, and erodes the foundation of overall happiness and contentment. As such, chronic inflammation emerges not only as a physical ailment but also as a formidable adversary to the preservation of mental and emotional well-being, as it casts a shadow over the prospect of leading a fulfilling and enriching life.

INFLAMMATION AND DEPRESSION

Exploring the relationship between inflammation and depression reveals an interplay that significantly influences overall QOL. Chronic inflammation—characterized by its persistent and dysregulated immune responses—has been implicated in the development and exacerbation of depressive symptoms. The inflammatory cascade triggers alterations in neurotransmitter activity, particularly serotonin and dopamine— crucial for mood regulation. These neurochemical changes disrupt the balance within the brain, thus, contributing to the emergence of depressive symptoms such as persistent sadness, loss of interest in activities, and changes in sleep and appetite.

Moreover, the bidirectional nature of the inflammation-depression relationship creates a vicious cycle wherein inflammation exacerbates depressive symptoms; in turn, depression fuels inflammatory responses. The debilitating effects of depression compounded by the physical discomfort and fatigue associated with chronic inflammation further erode one's QOL. Individuals grappling with both conditions often find themselves navigating a maze of emotional distress, physical limitations, and diminished cognitive function, hence, making it challenging to engage fully in daily activities and maintain meaningful social connections (Beurel et al., 2020).

PROACTIVE MANAGEMENT IMPORTANCE

Understanding and managing chronic inflammation is crucial for maintaining long-term health and well-being. By recognizing the signs and symptoms of inflammation early on, individuals can take proactive steps to address underlying issues and prevent the development of chronic diseases.

Chronic inflammation is often referred to as a "silent" or "hidden" danger because it can persist for years without causing noticeable symptoms. Meanwhile, it may quietly damage tissues and organs setting the stage for the development of various health conditions such as heart disease, diabetes, arthritis, and even cancer. Therefore, being proactive in managing inflammation is essential for preventing these serious health consequences.

Similar to its connection to atherosclerosis, chronic inflammation is closely linked to insulin resistance and the development of DM2. By addressing inflammation early on, individuals can reduce their risk of developing these and other chronic diseases.

Moreover, chronic inflammation can have a profound impact on overall QOL by affecting energy levels, mood, sleep, and daily functioning. By managing inflammation effectively, individuals can experience improvements in their physical health, mental well-being, and overall vitality. This proactive approach not only helps prevent disease but also promotes optimal health and longevity.

One proactive strategy is to adopt a healthy lifestyle that includes regular physical activity, a balanced diet, stress management techniques, and adequate sleep. Regular exercise helps reduce inflammation, improve cardiovascular health, and boost mood and energy levels. Consuming a diet rich in anti-inflammatory foods such as fruits, vegetables, whole grains, and fatty fish can also help lower inflammation levels and support overall health.

Moreover, chronic stress can trigger inflammation and contribute to the development of various health conditions. Therefore, incorporating stress-reducing activities such as meditation, deep breathing exercises, yoga, or spending time in nature can help lower stress levels and promote relaxation.

Additionally, ensuring adequate sleep is crucial for reducing inflammation and supporting overall health. Poor sleep quality can exacerbate inflammation and increase the risk of chronic diseases. Therefore, practicing good sleep hygiene habits such as maintaining a consistent sleep schedule, creating a relaxing bedtime routine, and creating a comfortable sleep environment can help improve sleep quality and reduce inflammation.

Furthermore, regular monitoring of inflammation markers through blood tests and working closely with healthcare professionals can help individuals identify and address inflammation early on. By staying proactive in managing inflammation, you can take control of their health, reduce their risk of developing chronic diseases, and improve their overall QOL.

We will look more into these proactive strategies in detail later on in the upcoming chapters.

QUESTIONS TO PONDER ON

- Have you experienced persistent symptoms like fatigue, joint pain, or digestive issues that may be indicative of chronic inflammation?
- Are you aware of the potential impact of chronic inflammation on your long-term health and well-being?
- Have you noticed any patterns or triggers in your lifestyle or environment that may contribute to inflammation?
- Are you actively taking steps to manage stress, which can exacerbate inflammation?
- Do you prioritize a balanced diet rich in anti-inflammatory foods to support your body's natural defense mechanisms?
- Are you engaging in regular physical activity to promote circulation, reduce inflammation, and support overall health?
- Have you considered incorporating mindfulness practices into your daily routine to manage stress and promote relaxation?
- Are you getting enough quality sleep each night, thus, recognizing its crucial role in regulating inflammation and supporting immune function?

- Have you discussed your concerns about chronic inflammation with a healthcare professional to develop a personalized management plan?
- Are you committed to making lifestyle changes and adopting proactive strategies to mitigate the hidden dangers of chronic inflammation and improve your QOL?

KEY TAKEAWAYS

- Recognize the insidious nature of chronic inflammation and its potential impact on overall health and well-being.
- Understand the connection between chronic inflammation and various diseases including heart disease, diabetes, arthritis, and autoimmune disorders.
- Appreciate how chronic inflammation can impair daily functioning and QOL by affecting energy levels, mood, sleep, and overall vitality.
- Take proactive steps to mitigate the hidden dangers of chronic inflammation by managing stress, adopting a balanced diet, engaging in regular physical activity, prioritizing sleep, and seeking professional guidance when needed.
- Embrace holistic approaches to inflammation management by incorporating mindfulness practices, dietary changes, and lifestyle modifications to support long-term health and vitality.

Our next destination is Chapter 3, where we explore how to recognize the signs and symptoms of chronic inflammation in ourselves and others, therefore, empowering ourselves to take proactive steps towards better health.

CHAPTER 3

IDENTIFYING CHRONIC INFLAMMATION

If you don't think your anxiety, depression, sadness and stress impact your physical health, think again. All of these emotions trigger chemical reactions in your body, which can lead to inflammation and a weakened immune system. Learn how to cope, sweet friend. There will always be dark days.

- Kriss Carr

T he thing about chronic inflammation is its origin and development: It may be caused by almost anything and even be beyond our control. From dietary factors to environmental toxins and genetic predispositions, chronic inflammation can stealthily wreak havoc on our bodies, as it silently sows the seeds of disease and discomfort. Following, we embark on a journey of self-discovery, as we learn to recognize the subtle signs and symptoms of chronic inflammation that may be hiding in plain sight. Through understanding the common causes and diagnostic methods, we gain the power to identify and confront this silent adversary, thus, paving the way for a healthier, more vibrant future.

COMMON CAUSES

The causes of chronic inflammation are quite many, as mentioned above. Here are some of the most common causes.

DIETARY FACTORS

Dietary factors play a significant role in either fueling or mitigating chronic inflammation in the body. Certain foods, particularly those high in refined sugars, unhealthy fats, and processed ingredients, can trigger inflammatory responses.

- **Refined sugars:** Foods and beverages high in refined sugars such as soft drinks, candy, pastries, and sweetened snacks can lead to spikes in blood sugar levels and promote inflammation. Not only do they lack essential nutrients but they also contribute to insulin resistance leading to elevated blood sugar levels and increased inflammation.
- **Unhealthy fats:** Trans and saturated fats found in fried foods, processed snacks, and fatty cuts of meat can also fuel inflammation. Not only do they promote the production of pro-inflammatory chemicals in the body but also they interfere with the function of anti-inflammatory compounds, consequently exacerbating the inflammatory response.
- **Processed ingredients:** Processed foods often contain additives, preservatives, and artificial ingredients that can trigger immune reactions and inflammation in the body. Ingredients like high-fructose corn syrup, artificial sweeteners, and hydrogenated oils are commonly found in processed snacks, ready-to-eat meals, and fast-food items,

hence, contributing to chronic inflammation when consumed regularly.

- **Refined carbohydrates:** Foods made with refined grains like white bread, white rice, and pasta can cause inflammation due to their high glycemic index, which leads to rapid spikes in blood sugar levels. Their lack of fiber and essential nutrients contributes to chronic inflammation and metabolic dysfunction when consumed in excess.
- **Vegetable oils:** Vegetable oils like soybean, corn, and sunflower oil are high in omega-6 fatty acids, which can promote inflammation in the body when consumed in excess. These oils are commonly used in processed foods, fried foods, and restaurant meals, thus, contribute to an imbalance of omega-6 to omega-3 fatty acids and drive inflammation (Gunnars, 2018).

On the other hand, a diet rich in whole, nutrient-dense foods such as fruits, vegetables, whole grains, and lean proteins can help reduce inflammation and support overall health—more on these healthy dietary aspects in Chapter 10.

ENVIRONMENTAL TOXINS

Environmental toxins are substances found in the air, water, soil, and food that can disrupt the body's natural processes and contribute to chronic inflammation. These toxins include pollutants, chemicals, heavy metals, pesticides, and other harmful substances that we encounter in our everyday environment.

- **Air pollution:** Exposure to air pollutants such as particulate matter, ozone, nitrogen dioxide, and sulfur dioxide has been linked to increased inflammation in the body. Inhalation of these pollutants can trigger oxidative stress and inflammation in the respiratory system leading to conditions like asthma, bronchitis, and chronic obstructive pulmonary disease (COPD). Long-term exposure to air pollution has also been associated with systemic inflammation and an increased risk of cardiovascular diseases including heart attacks and strokes.

- **Water contaminants:** Contaminants in drinking water such as heavy metals like lead, mercury, and arsenic, as well as industrial chemicals like polychlorinated biphenyls (PCBs) and per- and polyfluoroalkyl substances (PFAS) can contribute to inflammation and adverse health effects. These contaminants can enter the body through ingestion, absorption, or inhalation, subsequently accumulating in tissues and organs and disrupting normal physiological functions. Chronic exposure to water contaminants has been linked to inflammation-related conditions like kidney disease, liver damage, and autoimmune disorders.

- **Food additives and pesticides:** Food additives, preservatives, artificial sweeteners, and pesticide residues found in processed and conventionally grown foods can also promote inflammation in the body. These chemicals may disrupt gut microbiota, impair immune function, and trigger inflammatory responses. Consuming foods treated with pesticides or contaminated with chemical additives can contribute to systemic inflammation and increase the risk of chronic diseases including cancer, obesity, and neurodegenerative disorders.

- **Household and personal care products:** Many household and personal care products contain harmful chemicals like phthalates, parabens, and synthetic fragrances that can disrupt hormone balance, immune function, and inflammatory pathways. These chemicals can be absorbed through the skin, inhaled as vapors, or ingested inadvertently, subsequently contributing to chronic inflammation and exacerbating existing health conditions.

Switching to natural, non-toxic alternatives for household cleaning products, cosmetics, and personal care items can help reduce exposure to inflammatory toxins and support overall health.

Here are some practical tips on reducing exposure to harmful environmental factors:

- **Improve indoor air quality:** Use air purifiers with high efficiency particulate air (HEPA) filters to remove pollutants and allergens from indoor air. Ventilate your home regularly by opening windows and doors to allow fresh air to circulate. Avoid smoking indoors and minimize the use of chemical-based cleaning products, air fresheners, and candles that can release harmful volatile organic compounds (VOCs) into the air.
- **Filter drinking water:** Use water filtration filters or systems to certified to remove specific pollutants like lead, chlorine, fluoride, and heavy metals from tap water. Avoid storing water in plastic containers, especially those made with bisphenol A (BPA) that can leach harmful chemicals into the water.
- **Eat organic and whole foods:** Opt for organic fruits, vegetables, meats, and dairy products whenever possible to minimize exposure to pesticides, herbicides, and synthetic fertilizers. Choose whole, unprocessed foods and limit consumption of processed and packaged foods containing artificial additives, preservatives, and synthetic ingredients.
- **Reduce Chemical Exposure:** Use natural, eco-friendly alternatives to conventional household cleaners, laundry detergents, and personal care products. Look for products labeled "green," "natural," or "biodegradable" that are free of toxic chemicals, fragrances, and dyes. Avoid products

containing phthalates, parabens, triclosan, and other potentially harmful ingredients.

- **Practice safe food handling:** Wash fruits and vegetables thoroughly before eating or cooking to remove pesticide residues and contaminants. Store food in glass or stainless steel containers instead of plastic containers to minimize exposure to plasticizers and other chemicals. Choose fresh, locally sourced foods whenever possible to reduce transportation-related emissions and support sustainable agriculture practices.

- **Limit exposure to electromagnetic fields:** Reduce exposure to electromagnetic fields (EMFs) from electronic devices like cell phones, laptops, Wi-Fi routers, and microwave ovens. Use wired connections instead of wireless connections whenever feasible. Keep electronic devices away from the body especially during sleep, and use EMF shielding products to reduce exposure to radiation.

- **Support environmental advocacy:** Get involved in local and national efforts to advocate for clean air, water, and soil. Support policies and initiatives that promote environmental protection, sustainable development, and renewable energy sources. Participate in community clean-up events, tree planting campaigns, and educational workshops to raise awareness about environmental issues and inspire positive change.

STRESS

When you experience stress—whether physical, emotional, or psychological—your body's stress response is triggered. This leads to the release of stress hormones like cortisol and adrenaline, which prepare your body to deal with the perceived threat or challenge.

While the stress response is essential for survival in acute situations, chronic or prolonged stress can dysregulate the immune system and contribute to chronic inflammation. Chronic stress can lead to persistent activation of the body's stress response resulting in elevated levels of stress hormones and inflammatory markers (Ravi et al., 2021).

Additionally, chronic stress can suppress immune function and impair the body's ability to regulate inflammation. This can lead to a state of chronic low-grade inflammation characterized by sustained activation of the immune system and increased production of inflammatory cytokines.

Chronic stress has been linked to the development and exacerbation of various inflammatory diseases including cardiovascular disease, autoimmune disorders, gastrointestinal disorders, and mental health conditions like depression and anxiety. Chronic inflammation, in turn, can further exacerbate stress-related symptoms and contribute to a vicious cycle of stress and inflammation.

Stress can also influence lifestyle factors that contribute to chronic inflammation such as poor dietary choices, sedentary behavior, inadequate sleep, and substance abuse. These lifestyle factors can exacerbate stress-related inflammation and increase the risk of developing chronic diseases.

In Chapter 5, we will look at strategies for stress management.

GENETIC PREDISPOSITIONS

Our genetic makeup plays a significant role in determining our susceptibility to chronic inflammation. Genetic variations or mutations in certain genes can affect how our immune system responds to external stimuli including pathogens, toxins, and environmental stressors. These genetic variations can influence the production of inflammatory cytokines, function of immune cells, and regulation of inflammatory pathways.

Certain inherited traits or genetic predispositions can increase the likelihood of developing chronic inflammatory conditions. For example, individuals with a family history of autoimmune diseases like RA, lupus, or IBD may have a higher risk of developing similar conditions due to shared genetic factors. Similarly, genetic predispositions to conditions like obesity, insulin resistance, and cardiovascular disease can also contribute to chronic inflammation.

It is important to note that genetic predispositions interact with environmental factors to influence the development of chronic inflammation. While genetics may predispose individuals to certain inflammatory conditions, environmental factors such as diet, lifestyle, exposure to toxins, and stress can trigger or exacerbate inflammation in genetically susceptible individuals. This concept of gene-environment interactions highlights the complex interplay between genetic and environmental factors in the pathogenesis of chronic inflammatory diseases.

Understanding the role of genetic predispositions in chronic inflammation has significant implications for personalized medicine and healthcare. Genetic testing and genomic analysis can help identify individuals at increased risk of developing inflammatory diseases and guide personalized treatment strategies. By targeting specific genetic pathways or risk factors, healthcare providers can tailor interventions to address the underlying causes of inflammation and improve patient outcomes.

SIGNS AND SYMPTOMS

Navigating the landscape of chronic inflammation requires a keen eye for the subtle cues that our bodies often provide. Unraveling the signs and symptoms of chronic inflammation equips us with the tools needed to identify and address this silent assailant.

LINGERING FATIGUE

Chronic inflammation—characterized by a prolonged and dysregulated immune response—often presents with lingering fatigue as one of its primary symptoms. This persistent exhaustion persists despite sufficient rest and sleep, thus, impacting an individuals' ability to engage in daily activities and reducing their overall well-being.

The fatigue associated with chronic inflammation is more than just feeling tired; it is a profound and pervasive sense of weariness that pervades every aspect of life. Individuals may wake up feeling unrefreshed, struggle to concentrate or focus throughout the day, and find even simple tasks exhausting.

This constant state of fatigue can have far-reaching consequences affecting not only physical energy levels but also mental and emotional well-being. It may lead to decreased productivity at work or school, strained relationships due to limited energy for social interactions, and feelings of frustration or hopelessness about the inability to overcome the exhaustion.

Furthermore, the relentless nature of chronic fatigue can exacerbate existing health conditions and make it challenging to pursue healthy lifestyle habits. Physical exercise, which is essential for managing inflammation, may feel daunting or impossible when every movement requires monumental effort. Similarly, maintaining a nutritious diet may become a struggle when fatigue saps the motivation to prepare meals or make healthy food choices.

JOINT PAIN AND STIFFNESS

Inflammation affecting the joints can result in a range of symptoms including pain, stiffness, and reduced mobility. Individuals may notice discomfort in their joints, which often intensifies with movement, thus, hindering their ability to carry out everyday tasks.

Joint pain associated with inflammation is typically characterized by a dull, aching sensation that may be localized to specific joints or spread throughout the body. This pain can vary in severity ranging from mild discomfort to sharp, stabbing sensations that significantly impact mobility and QOL.

Stiffness is another common symptom of joint inflammation particularly noticeable after periods of inactivity or upon waking in the morning. Individuals may find it challenging to bend or flex their joints fully, as they experience a sensation of tightness or resistance with movement.

The decreased range of motion accompanying joint inflammation further complicates daily activities, as individuals may struggle to perform simple tasks such as reaching, bending, or walking comfortably. Activities that require repetitive or weight-bearing movements such as climbing stairs or lifting objects may exacerbate joint pain and stiffness, hence, further limiting functionality.

DIGESTIVE ISSUES

Chronic inflammation can disrupt normal gastrointestinal function leading to a range of digestive issues that affect overall well-being. Individuals may experience symptoms reflecting an imbalance in gut health and inflammatory processes, such as bloating, abdominal pain, diarrhea, or constipation.

Bloating is a common complaint associated with inflammation in the digestive system characterized by a sensation of fullness or tightness in the abdomen. This uncomfortable swelling may occur after meals or persist throughout the day often accompanied by increased gas production and discomfort.

Abdominal pain is another hallmark symptom of gastrointestinal inflammation manifesting as cramping, sharp or dull pain, or discomfort in the stomach region. Its severity and duration may vary ranging from mild and intermittent to severe and persistent, subsequently impacting daily activities and well-being.

Changes in bowel habits are also indicative of digestive inflammation with individuals experiencing alterations in stool frequency, consistency, or texture. Diarrhea and constipation characterized by loose or watery stools and infrequent or difficult bowel movements, respectively, are common manifestations of gastrointestinal inflammation.

These digestive disturbances can disrupt normal bowel function leading to discomfort, inconvenience, and embarrassment. Moreover, they may impact nutritional absorption, thereby impairing the body's ability to extract essential nutrients from food and maintain optimal health.

SKIN PROBLEMS

Inflammation can have visible effects on the skin presenting as redness, swelling, itching, or rashes. Skin conditions such as eczema, psoriasis, or acne often worsen due to underlying inflammatory processes.

Atopic dermatitis—most commonly referred to as eczema—is characterized by red, itchy patches on the skin that may ooze or crust over. These flare-ups result from an inflammatory response triggered by various factors including allergens, irritants, or stressors.

Psoriasis is another chronic skin condition characterized by thick, red patches covered with silvery scales. It occurs when the immune system mistakenly attacks healthy skin cells leading to rapid turnover and the formation of plaques. Inflammation plays a central role in the pathogenesis of psoriasis, as it drives the excessive growth and accumulation of skin cells.

Acne—a common skin disorder—results from inflammation of the hair follicles and sebaceous glands. It presents as pimples, blackheads, whiteheads, or cysts on the face, chest, back, or other areas of the body. Inflammatory mediators released by immune cells contribute to the development of acne lesions, hence, exacerbating the condition.

Inflammatory skin problems not only cause physical discomfort but also impact emotional well-being and self-esteem. Individuals may experience embarrassment, frustration, or anxiety due to the visible effects of inflammation on their skin. Moreover, persistent inflammation can lead to scarring, hyperpigmentation, or other long-term complications further affecting skin health and appearance.

PERSISTENT HEADACHES

Persistent headaches are another common symptom of chronic inflammation, which can contribute to recurrent headaches or migraines. Individuals experiencing chronic inflammation may frequently suffer from headaches characterized by throbbing pain, pressure, or tightness in the head. These headaches can vary in intensity and duration, ranging from mild discomfort to debilitating pain that interferes with daily activities.

Chronic inflammation can trigger headaches through various mechanisms including the release of inflammatory mediators that sensitize pain receptors in the brain and blood vessels. Additionally, inflammation in the blood vessels surrounding the brain may lead to vasodilation or constriction contributing to headache development.

Individuals with chronic inflammation may also experience associated symptoms such as sensitivity to light or sound, nausea, and fatigue during headache episodes. These symptoms can further impair daily productivity and standard of living, thereby affecting mood, concentration, and overall well-being.

MUSCLE WEAKNESS

Muscle weakness is another prevalent symptom of chronic inflammation characterized by reduced strength, endurance, and coordination in affected individuals. Chronic inflammation can lead to the breakdown of muscle tissue and impair the normal functioning of muscles resulting in weakness and fatigue.

Individuals experiencing inflammation-induced muscle weakness may notice difficulty performing physical tasks or engaging in exercise due to decreased muscle strength and endurance. Simple activities such as lifting objects, climbing stairs, or walking long distances may become challenging and exhausting.

Inflammation can disrupt the normal signaling pathways that control muscle contraction and relaxation leading to impaired muscle function. Additionally, inflammatory mediators released during chronic inflammation can directly damage muscle cells and interfere with their ability to generate force efficiently.

Muscle weakness associated with chronic inflammation can have a significant impact on daily functioning and livability. It may limit individuals' ability to participate in activities they enjoy, affect their independence, and contribute to feelings of frustration and decreased self-esteem.

COGNITIVE IMPAIRMENT

Cognitive impairment is another consequence of chronic inflammation affecting various aspects of mental function such as memory, concentration, and mental clarity. Chronic inflammation can disrupt normal brain function leading to cognitive difficulties that can significantly impact daily life.

Individuals experiencing cognitive impairment due to chronic inflammation may notice symptoms such as memory lapses, difficulty concentrating on tasks, or a feeling of mental fog. These cognitive challenges can interfere with work or academic performance, impair decision-making abilities, and affect overall productivity and QOL

The inflammatory processes associated with chronic inflammation can directly affect the structure and function of the brain leading to alterations in neurotransmitter activity, neuronal communication, and synaptic plasticity. These changes can contribute to cognitive dysfunction and impairments in cognitive processes such as learning, memory formation, and information processing.

Furthermore, chronic inflammation can exacerbate underlying neurological conditions such as Alzheimer's disease, Parkinson's disease, or multiple sclerosis leading to accelerated cognitive decline and worsening symptoms. Inflammatory mediators released during chronic inflammation can contribute to neurodegenerative processes, neuronal damage, and the formation of amyloid plaques and neurofibrillary tangles in the brain.

MOOD CHANGES

Chronic inflammation can have a significant impact on mood regulation leading to changes in emotional well-being and mental health. Individuals experiencing chronic inflammation may notice symptoms of depression, anxiety, or irritability, which can affect their overall mood.

The inflammatory processes associated with chronic inflammation can disrupt the balance of neurotransmitters in the brain including serotonin, dopamine, and norepinephrine, which play key roles in regulating mood and emotions. Imbalances in these neurotransmitters can contribute to the development of mood disorders such as depression and anxiety.

In addition, chronic inflammation can activate stress pathways in the brain, therefore, increase the production of stress hormones such as cortisol. Elevated levels of cortisol can further exacerbate mood disturbances contributing to feelings of anxiety, tension, and emotional instability.

Moreover, the hypothalamic-pituitary-adrenal (HPA) axis—a key system involved in the body's stress response—can also succumb to chronic inflammation. Dysregulation of the HPA axis can lead to abnormalities in cortisol secretion, which may contribute to mood disorders and exacerbate symptoms of depression and anxiety.

Individuals experiencing mood changes due to chronic inflammation may also notice alterations in sleep patterns, appetite, and energy levels further impacting their overall mental health and well-being. These mood disturbances can interfere with daily functioning, relationships, and the overall QOL.

RECURRENT INFECTIONS

Chronic inflammation can compromise the immune system leaving individuals vulnerable to recurrent infections. This heightened inflammatory state can weaken the body's defense mechanisms making it easier for pathogens such as bacteria, viruses, and fungi to invade and proliferate.

When the immune system is chronically activated, it can become overworked and less efficient at recognizing and fighting off infections. As a result, individuals may experience more frequent bouts of illness including colds, flu, sinus infections, urinary tract infections, and other common infections.

The inflammatory processes associated with chronic inflammation can disrupt the normal function of immune cells, such as white blood cells, which play a crucial role in identifying and destroying pathogens. Additionally, chronic inflammation can impair the production of antibodies—proteins that help the immune system recognize and neutralize invading microorganisms.

Moreover, chronic inflammation can create an environment within the body supportive of microbial growth and proliferation. Inflammatory mediators released during chronic inflammation can promote the survival and replication of pathogens, thus, further exacerbating the risk of infection.

Individuals experiencing recurrent infections may notice symptoms such as fever, cough, sore throat, fatigue, and malaise. These infections can be particularly challenging to manage, as the body may struggle to mount an effective immune response due to underlying inflammatory dysfunction.

UNEXPLAINED WEIGHT CHANGES

Chronic inflammation can disrupt the body's metabolic processes leading to unexplained fluctuations in weight. In fact, it can interfere with the normal regulation of metabolism, which includes processes such as energy expenditure, nutrient absorption, and fat storage. As a result, individuals may suddenly gain or lose body weight despite maintaining consistent dietary and exercise routines.

In cases of chronic inflammation, the body may produce inflammatory molecules that affect hormones involved in metabolism such as insulin and leptin. These hormones play crucial roles in regulating appetite, energy balance, and fat storage. Dysregulation of these hormones due to inflammation can lead to abnormal changes in body weight.

For example, chronic inflammation may contribute to insulin resistance i.e., elevated blood sugar levels and increased fat storage due to the cells reduced responsiveness to insulin resulting in weight gain, particularly around the abdomen.

Conversely, inflammation-induced alterations in leptin signaling can disrupt the body's ability to regulate appetite and energy expenditure leading to decreased food intake and unintentional weight loss. Inflammatory processes may also stimulate the breakdown of muscle tissue further contributing to weight loss.

Unexplained weight changes due to chronic inflammation can have significant implications for overall health and well-being. Excess weight gain is associated with an increased risk of metabolic disorders such as DM2, cardiovascular disease, and fatty liver disease. On the other hand, unintended weight loss can indicate underlying health issues and may lead to nutritional deficiencies and muscle wasting.

DIAGNOSTIC METHODS AND MEDICAL TESTS

The first step in identifying chronic inflammation is to recognize the signs and symptoms that may indicate its presence. However, to confirm a diagnosis of chronic inflammation and understand its underlying causes, medical tests and diagnostic methods are essential.

Medical professionals use a variety of tests and procedures to assess inflammation levels in the body and pinpoint potential sources of inflammation. These diagnostic methods help to gather valuable information about the extent and nature of inflammation, subsequently guiding appropriate treatment strategies.

One common diagnostic tool used to assess inflammation is blood tests, which measure markers of inflammation in the bloodstream. These markers include C-reactive protein (CRP), erythrocyte sedimentation rate (ESR), and pro-inflammatory cytokines. Elevated levels of these markers may indicate the presence of inflammation and provide insights into its severity.

Additionally, imaging studies such as X-rays, ultrasound, magnetic resonance imaging (MRI), and computed tomography (CT) scans allow healthcare professionals to visualize and identify areas of inflammation and assess tissue damage associated with chronic inflammation such as joint damage in arthritis or organ involvement in autoimmune diseases.

In some cases, specialized tests may be ordered to evaluate specific aspects of inflammation or assess organ function. For example, endoscopic procedures such as colonoscopy or endoscopy may be performed to examine the gastrointestinal tract for signs of inflammation in conditions like IBD. Biopsy samples may also be collected from affected tissues for further analysis under a microscope.

It is important for you to be proactive in learning about these diagnostic methods and discussing them with your healthcare providers. By understanding the available tests and procedures, you can actively participate in your healthcare journey and advocate for appropriate diagnostic evaluations when necessary. Early detection and accurate diagnosis of chronic inflammation are crucial for initiating timely treatment and preventing complications associated with inflammatory conditions.

QUESTIONS TO PONDER ON

- Are there any specific dietary habits or environmental factors that you suspect may be contributing to inflammation in your body?
- Have you experienced any recent changes in your overall health or well-being that warrant further investigation for chronic inflammation?
- Are you aware of the potential impact of chronic inflammation on your long-term health and QOL?
- Have you discussed your concerns about chronic inflammation with your healthcare provider, and if not, do

you plan to bring it up during your next appointment?

- Are you interested in learning more about diagnostic tests and procedures that can help assess inflammation levels and identify potential sources of inflammation in your body?
- Have you considered making any lifestyle modifications, such as changes to your diet or stress management techniques, to help reduce inflammation and improve your overall health?
- Are you willing to take proactive steps to address any underlying inflammation and optimize your health and well-being?
- Are you committed to staying informed and empowered as you navigate the journey of identifying and managing chronic inflammation for long-term health and vitality?

As we delve deeper into understanding the relationship between our gut and immune system, we embark on a transformative journey toward optimizing our health. In Chapter 4, we unravel the mysteries of the gut-immune connection and explore the profound impact of gut health on our overall well-being.

CHAPTER 4

GUT-IMMUNE CONNECTION AND GUT HEALTH

Reduce inflammation to treat the root of many issues. If your gut isn't working right, it can cause so many other issues.

- Jay Woodman

The intriguing concept of the gut as our second brain highlights the profound influence that your gut health can have on your overall well-being. In this chapter, we will dive into the fascinating world of the gut-immune connection by exploring the intimate connection between your gut health, immune system, and systemic inflammation.

THE GUT-INFLAMMATORY AXIS

The gut-inflammatory axis refers to the constant interplay between your gut health and inflammation. Think of it as a feedback loop where the state of your gut influences the level of inflammation in your body; inflammation, in turn, can impact your gut's health.

Your gastrointestinal tract aka gut houses trillions of bacteria, fungi, and other microorganisms collectively known as the gut microbiota that play a crucial role in maintaining gut health by aiding in digestion, nutrient absorption, and immune function. When their balance is disrupted, it can lead to gut dysbiosis—a condition associated with inflammation.

Dysbiosis and gut inflammation can lead to the leakage of bacterial toxins and other harmful molecules from the gut into the bloodstream—a phenomenon known as leaky gut syndrome. These toxins can trigger an immune response throughout the body leading to systemic inflammation. Systemic inflammation has been implicated in the development and progression of various chronic diseases.

Conversely, systemic inflammation can also influence your gut health. Chronic inflammation can disrupt the gut lining leading to increased intestinal permeability i.e., "leaky gut." When the gut barrier is compromised, it allows toxins, bacteria, and undigested food particles to enter the bloodstream further fueling inflammation and perpetuating the cycle.

GUT MICROBIOME

These microorganisms play essential roles in maintaining your health. They help break down food, produce vitamins, and regulate your immune system. Furthermore, they interact with the cells lining your gut, thus, influencing various physiological processes.

The diversity and composition of your gut microbiome are influenced by factors such as diet, lifestyle, medications, and environmental exposures. A healthy gut microbiome is characterized by a rich variety of microbial species—each performing specific functions to support your well-being.

A balanced and diverse gut microbiome is crucial for maintaining optimal health and well-being. Just like a thriving ecosystem in nature, a diverse microbiome ensures stability and resilience against disturbances.

A healthy gut microbiome helps to:

- **Support digestive health:** Beneficial microbes aid in breaking down food, fermenting fibers, and producing essential nutrients like vitamins B and K. They also help maintain the integrity of the gut lining, hence, preventing leaky gut and digestive disorders.
- **Regulate immune function:** The gut microbiome plays a vital role in training and modulating the immune system. By interacting with immune cells in the gut-associated lymphoid tissue (GALT), beneficial microbes help to distinguish between harmful pathogens and harmless antigens, thus, preventing inappropriate immune responses.
- **Protect against pathogens:** Beneficial microbes compete with harmful pathogens for nutrients and space in the gut, crowd out potential invaders, and reduce the risk of infections.
- **Influence brain health:** The gut microbiome communicates with the brain through the gut-brain axis influencing mood, cognition, and behavior. A healthy gut microbiome is associated with reduced risk of mood disorders like depression and anxiety.
- **Maintain metabolic health:** Certain microbes in the gut play a role in regulating metabolism and energy balance. A balanced microbiome is associated with a lower risk of metabolic disorders such as obesity, DM2, and cardiovascular disease.

LEAKY GUT SYNDROME

Leaky gut syndrome, scientifically known as increased intestinal permeability, is a condition where the lining of the small intestine becomes damaged, therefore, allowing undigested food particles, toxins, and microbes to leak into the bloodstream. Normally, the cells lining the intestinal wall are tightly packed together forming a barrier that regulates the passage of nutrients and other substances into the bloodstream. However, various factors such as chronic inflammation, stress, poor diet, medications, and infections can compromise the integrity of this barrier leading to gaps or "leaks" between the cells.

When the intestinal barrier is compromised, harmful substances that would typically be kept out of the bloodstream can enter freely. This triggers an immune response as the body perceives these substances as foreign invaders, subsequently leading to inflammation and potential immune system over-activation.

Common symptoms of leaky gut syndrome may include digestive issues such as bloating, gas, diarrhea, or constipation, as well as food sensitivities, fatigue, headaches, skin problems, and joint pain. However, it is essential to note that leaky gut syndrome is a complex and multifactorial condition, and its diagnosis and treatment may require a comprehensive approach that addresses underlying factors contributing to intestinal permeability.

Increased intestinal permeability disrupts the barrier function of the intestinal lining, allowing unwanted substances to pass through into the bloodstream. This breach in the gut barrier can lead to systemic inflammation as the immune system responds to the presence of these foreign invaders. Normally, the intestinal lining acts as a protective barrier selectively allowing nutrients to be absorbed while preventing harmful substances like bacteria, toxins, and undigested food particles from entering the bloodstream. However, when the integrity of this barrier is compromised—as in leaky gut syndrome—

these substances can leak through the gaps between the cells lining the intestines.

Once in the bloodstream, these foreign substances trigger an immune response leading to the release of pro-inflammatory cytokines and other immune mediators. This systemic inflammation can have far-reaching effects throughout the body contributing to the development or exacerbation of various inflammatory conditions and chronic diseases. Additionally, the presence of inflammatory cytokines in the bloodstream can further disrupt the integrity of the gut barrier, hence, creating a vicious cycle of inflammation and intestinal permeability.

In this way, increased intestinal permeability can perpetuate inflammation both locally in the gut and systemically throughout the body. Addressing leaky gut syndrome and restoring gut barrier function is therefore crucial for mitigating inflammation and promoting overall health and well-being.

PROBIOTICS, PREBIOTICS, AND GUT-FRIENDLY FOODS

Probiotics are live microorganisms that, when consumed in adequate amounts, confer health benefits to the host. Prebiotics, on the other hand, are non-digestible fibers that serve as food for probiotics and other beneficial bacteria in the gut.

Probiotics can be found in fermented foods such as yogurt, kefir, sauerkraut, and kimchi, as well as in dietary supplements. These live cultures replenish the gut with beneficial bacteria, thus, maintain microbial balance and support digestion. Prebiotics are abundant in foods like garlic, onions, bananas, asparagus, and whole grains. By incorporating both probiotic-rich and prebiotic-containing foods into your diet, you can optimize gut health and promote the growth of beneficial bacteria.

Probiotics and prebiotics have garnered attention for their potential to modulate inflammation and promote a healthy gut microbiome. Probiotics restore microbial balance and diversity by introducing beneficial bacteria into the gut, which is essential for immune function and inflammation regulation. These live microorganisms can interact with the immune system and produce anti-inflammatory compounds, thereby reducing inflammation and supporting gut health.

Prebiotics, on the other hand, serve as fuel for probiotics and other beneficial bacteria in the gut. By nourishing these microbes, prebiotics promote their growth and activity, thus, maintain a diverse and resilient gut microbiome. This, in turn, contributes to a balanced immune response and can help alleviate inflammation. Additionally, prebiotics have been shown to enhance the production of short-chain fatty acids, which have anti-inflammatory properties and play a crucial role in gut health (Markowiak & Śliżewska, 2017).

STRATEGIES FOR IMPROVING GUT HEALTH

Encompassing a range of approaches aimed at promoting a balanced and thriving gut microbiome, one key strategy involves incorporating fibrous foods into your diet. This entails focusing on consuming a variety of fiber-rich foods such as fruits, vegetables, whole grains, legumes, and nuts. Fiber serves as fuel for beneficial gut bacteria, therefore, promoting their growth and diversity. Aim to include both soluble and insoluble fiber in your diet to support digestive health and regular bowel movements.

Diversifying your diet to include a wide range of nutrient sources is another crucial aspect of improving gut health. This means incorporating foods rich in lean proteins, healthy fats, vitamins, and minerals. Antioxidant-rich foods, such as berries, leafy greens, and nuts can help combat oxidative stress and inflammation. Opting for whole, minimally processed foods maximizes nutrient intake and supports overall health.

Integrating probiotics and prebiotics into your diet is also essential for promoting gut health. Probiotic-rich foods like yogurt, kefir, sauerkraut, and kimchi introduce beneficial bacteria into the gut. Meanwhile, prebiotic-containing foods such as garlic, onions, bananas, and asparagus provide nourishment for probiotics and support their growth.

Moreover, it is crucial to prioritize adequate hydration by consuming plenty of water throughout the day, as it plays a significant role in maintaining gut health. Limiting the intake of dehydrating beverages like sugary sodas, caffeinated drinks, and alcohol can help maintain optimal hydration levels and support digestive function.

In addition to staying hydrated, practicing mindful eating habits can further enhance gut health. Mindful eating involves paying attention to the sensations of hunger and fullness, as well as being aware of the taste, texture, and aroma of food. By slowing down during meals, chewing food thoroughly, and savoring each bite, you can improve digestion and nutrient absorption while reducing the likelihood of overeating or digestive discomfort. Incorporating mindfulness into your eating routine can also help reduce stress levels, which is beneficial for overall gut health.

Slow and conscious eating involves taking the time to fully engage with your meals, savoring each bite, and being mindful of the eating process. By eating slowly, you give your body a chance to properly digest food and signal feelings of fullness, which can prevent overeating and promote better digestion.

Being aware of food triggers—such as certain ingredients or types of food that may cause discomfort or inflammation in the gut—can help you make informed dietary choices to support gut health. By paying attention to how your body responds to different foods, you can tailor your diet to better suit your individual needs and preferences, ultimately promoting a healthier gut microbiome.

QUESTIONS TO PONDER ON

- How can you incorporate more probiotic and prebiotic-rich foods into your diet to support gut health?
- What mindful eating practices can you adopt to improve digestion and reduce inflammation?
- Are you aware of any food triggers that may exacerbate gut-related symptoms or inflammation?
- What strategies can you implement to promote slow and conscious eating habits in your daily routine?
- Have you considered the role of fiber in your diet and how it can benefit gut health?
- What steps can you take to diversify your nutrient sources and ensure a well-rounded diet for optimal gut function?
- Are there any lifestyle changes you can make to reduce stress and support a healthier gut-immune connection?

As we conclude our exploration of gut health and its profound impact on inflammation, we now turn our attention to another crucial factor in the inflammatory process: stress. Chapter 5 delves into the relationship between stress and inflammation by shedding light on how our emotional well-being can influence our body's inflammatory responses.

CHAPTER 5
STRESS AND INFLAMMATION

He snapped the notebook shut. "I know all of this must be very frightening for you, but try not to agitate yourself. Excitement will only worsen the inflammation."

- Margaret Rogerson.

In today's world, stress has become an unavoidable part of our lives, but did you know that it could be silently fueling inflammation within your body? As we navigate the complexities of modern life, our bodies often respond to stressors by triggering an inflammatory response, consequently setting the stage for chronic inflammation and a host of related health issues.

CONNECTION BETWEEN STRESS, CORTISOL LEVELS, AND INFLAMMATION

Stress is the body's natural response to demands or pressures from the environment. It can be triggered by various both positive and negative situations or events that require us to adapt or respond.

Stress can manifest as physical, emotional, or psychological tension, and it often involves a complex interplay of physiological and psychological processes. While acute stress can be beneficial in helping us deal with immediate challenges, chronic or prolonged stress can have detrimental effects on our health and well-being.

Think of your body as having a built-in security system. Stress acts like the alarm that activates when there is a threat. Initially; this alarm helps us react promptly to danger. However, if it continues to sound off constantly, it can strain the system and result in issues such as inflammation. When our stress response remains chronically activated, inflammation can persist in our bodies even in the absence of an actual threat.

Stress triggers a cascade of physiological responses in the body primarily orchestrated by the release of cortisol and other stress hormones. Initially, this response is adaptive, preparing the body to confront or flee from perceived threats—a mechanism often referred to as the "fight or flight" response.

During acute stress, cortisol mobilizes energy reserves, sharpens focus, and enhances physical performance allowing individuals to effectively cope with immediate challenges. However, chronic or persistent stress can lead to sustained elevations of cortisol levels, thereby disrupting the intricate balance of the immune system.

Cortisol exerts its effects on immune function by interacting with immune cells and modulating their activity. In the short term, cortisol can suppress certain aspects of the immune response, such as inflammation, to divert resources toward immediate survival needs. However, chronic exposure to elevated cortisol levels can dysregulate immune function leading to immune system dysfunction and increased susceptibility to inflammation (Morey et al., 2015).

Stress-induced alterations in immune function can disrupt the balance between pro- and anti-inflammatory processes tipping the scale towards chronic inflammation. This chronic inflammatory state is associated with a myriad of adverse health outcomes including cardiovascular disease, metabolic disorders, autoimmune conditions, and mental health disorders.

Moreover, stress can also influence our behaviors and lifestyle choices like reaching for comfort foods high in sugar and unhealthy fats, which can further contribute to inflammation. Additionally, stress can disrupt our sleep patterns, weaken our immune system, and affect our digestive health, all of which play roles in inflammation.

STRATEGIES FOR MANAGING STRESS

Managing stress is crucial for your overall health and well-being. By adopting effective stress management techniques, you can experience a multitude of benefits that positively impact your life.

Firstly, managing stress can make you feel happier and more relaxed. This reduction in stress levels contributes to a healthier body overall, as chronic stress has been linked to various health issues such as heart disease and weakened immune function. You will also notice that you have a clearer mind and improved cognitive function allowing you to think more clearly and focus better on the tasks at hand.

Additionally, effective stress management techniques can enhance your relationships with others. You will find that you are better equipped to communicate and handle conflicts without being overwhelmed by stress. You will also have increased energy levels providing you with the vitality needed to engage in activities you enjoy and tackle daily challenges with vigor.

Better sleep is another notable benefit of stress management. Reduced stress levels can lead to improved sleep quality and duration, ultimately contributing to your overall well-being. By effectively managing stress, you will be better equipped to handle problems and adversities that arise in life, as you will not be consumed by overwhelming stress responses.

Better stress management is not only crucial for your mental and emotional well-being but also plays a significant role in managing inflammation in your body. When you are under chronic stress, your body produces high levels of cortisol—the stress hormone—which can trigger inflammatory responses. Persistent inflammatory responses can lead to chronic inflammation contributing to various health problems such as heart disease, diabetes, and autoimmune conditions.

Incorporating stress management strategies into your daily routine is essential for maintaining optimal health and preventing the detrimental effects of chronic inflammation. By taking proactive steps to manage stress, you can support your body's natural ability to regulate inflammation and promote overall well-being.

MINDFULNESS

Mindfulness is a practice that involves being fully present and aware of the present moment without judgment. It entails paying attention to thoughts, feelings, bodily sensations, and the surrounding environment with openness and acceptance. In the context of stress reduction, mindfulness helps individuals become more attuned to their internal experiences and external surroundings, hence, allows them to respond to stressors with greater clarity and resilience.

The principles of mindfulness include cultivating non-judgmental awareness, which involves observing thoughts and emotions without labelling them as good or bad. It also involves practicing acceptance, acknowledging, and allowing experiences to unfold without resistance. Additionally, mindfulness emphasizes living in the present moment, letting go of worries about the past or future, and focusing attention on the here and now.

- **Start with short sessions**: Begin with brief mindfulness sessions such as 5–10 min of mindful breathing. Gradually increase the duration as you become more comfortable with the practice.
- **Set reminders**: Use cues throughout your day to remind yourself to be mindful. This could be a recurring alarm on your phone, sticky note on your desk, or visual cue like a specific object or photo.
- **Practice mindful eating**: Pay attention to the taste, texture, and sensations of each bite when eating. Chew slowly and savor the flavors while noticing how food nourishes your body and brings pleasure to the present moment.
- **Take mindful breaks**: Incorporate short mindfulness breaks into your daily routine. Pause for a few moments to focus on your breath, observe your surroundings, or check in with how you are feeling physically and emotionally.
- **Use everyday activities as opportunities**: Turn routine activities like washing dishes, showering, or walking into opportunities for mindfulness. Focus on the sensations, movements, and sounds involved in each task, thus, bringing your full attention to the present moment.
- **Practice gratitude**: Take time each day to reflect on things you are grateful for. This can be done through journaling, mental reflection, or simply pausing to appreciate the blessings in your life.
- **Engage fully in activities**: When engaging in activities, give them your full attention and immerse yourself in the experience. Whether it is reading, exercising, or spending time with loved ones, be present and engaged in the moment.
- **Cultivate self-compassion**: Approach yourself with kindness and understanding, especially during challenging

moments. Treat yourself with the same compassion you would offer to a friend facing difficulties.

MEDITATION

Meditation is a practice that involves training the mind to achieve a state of focused attention, relaxation, and heightened awareness. It encompasses various techniques and approaches aimed at cultivating mental clarity, emotional balance, and inner peace. Through meditation, individuals cultivate a deeper understanding of themselves as they observe their thoughts, feelings and experiences without judgment.

Mindfulness and meditation often go hand in hand complementing each other in the pursuit of mental and emotional well-being. While mindfulness emphasizes present-moment awareness and acceptance of one's thoughts and feelings, meditation provides a structured practice for cultivating mindfulness and enhancing self-awareness. Together, these practices offer powerful tools for managing stress, reducing anxiety, and promoting overall mental resilience.

MINDFULNESS MEDITATION

Mindfulness meditation involves focusing on the present moment without judgment and observing thoughts, sensations, and emotions as they arise.

Mindfulness meditation helps reduce stress by promoting relaxation, calming the mind, and fostering resilience to stressors. It also has been shown to lower inflammation levels in the body by reducing cortisol production and modulating the immune response.

Approach

- Find a quiet and comfortable space to sit or lie down.

- Close your eyes gently.
- Focus your attention on your breath.
- Allow thoughts to come and go without judgment.
- Notice any sensations in your body.
- Pay attention to the sounds in your environment.
- Bring your attention back to your breath whenever your mind wanders.
- Continue this practice for a few minutes gradually increasing the duration as you feel more comfortable.

LOVING-KINDNESS MEDITATION

Loving-kindness meditation is a practice aimed at fostering feelings of compassion, kindness, and goodwill towards oneself and others. It involves directing positive intentions and well-wishes towards oneself, loved ones, acquaintances, and even individuals with whom you may have difficulties. This meditation encourages a sense of interconnectedness and empathy, hence, promoting emotional resilience and strengthening social bonds.

Loving-kindness meditation promotes emotional well-being, reduces negative emotions such as anger and resentment, and fosters social connections. By enhancing positive emotions, it can buffer against the harmful effects of stress and inflammation.

Approach

- Start by finding a quiet and comfortable space to sit or lie down.
- Close your eyes and take a few deep breaths to center yourself.
- Begin by directing loving-kindness towards yourself. Silently repeat phrases like "May I be happy, may I be healthy, may I be safe, may I live with ease."

- Visualize yourself surrounded by warmth and love as you repeat these phrases.
- Once you feel a sense of kindness towards yourself, extend these wishes to loved ones silently repeating similar phrases for them.
- Gradually, extend these feelings of loving-kindness to acquaintances, strangers, and even individuals you may have difficulties with.
- Maintain a sense of openness and compassion as you cultivate these feelings towards yourself and others.
- Take a few moments to reflect on the experience and notice any shifts in your emotions or mindset.

GUIDED IMAGERY

Guided imagery is a relaxation technique that involves creating vivid mental images of peaceful and calming scenes or scenarios. These visualizations are designed to evoke feelings of relaxation, calmness, and positive emotions. During guided imagery exercises, you are guided through a series of detailed descriptions of calming environments, such as serene natural settings, tranquil beaches, or lush forests. By immersing yourself in these mental images, you can experience a sense of escape from stress and tension allowing your minds and bodies to relax deeply. Guided imagery can be accompanied by soothing music or calming narration to enhance the overall relaxation experience.

Guided imagery induces a state of deep relaxation, therefore, reducing stress hormones and promoting feelings of well-being. It can also enhance immune function and decrease inflammation by activating the body's relaxation response.

Approach

- Find a comfortable position in a quiet environment.

- Listen to a guided imagery recording or read a guided imagery script.
- Close your eyes and focus on your breath to relax.
- Visualize yourself in a serene and tranquil environment, such as a peaceful beach or a serene forest.
- Use all your senses to vividly experience the sights, sounds, and sensations of the scene.
- Allow to fully immerse yourself in the mental imagery and let go of any tension or stress.

ESTABLISHING A MEDITATION ROUTINE

Integrate meditation into your daily routine until it becomes a natural habit just like brushing your teeth or exercising. Consistency is key to experiencing the long-term benefits of meditation on stress resilience and inflammation reduction.

- **Start small:** Begin with short meditation sessions, even just 5–10 min a day, and gradually increase the duration as you become more comfortable.
- **Choose a convenient time:** Select a time of day that works best for you, whether it is in the morning before starting your day, during a lunch break, or in the evening before bedtime.
- **Create a dedicated space:** Designate a quiet and comfortable area in your home where you can meditate without distractions. This could be a corner of a room or a cozy spot with cushions and soft lighting.
- **Set realistic goals:** Instead of aiming for perfection, focus on consistency. Set achievable goals for yourself, such as meditating for a certain number of days per week or increasing your meditation duration gradually.
- **Use guided meditations:** Utilize guided meditation apps, podcasts, or online resources to help you get started and

stay focused during your meditation practice.

- **Stay patient and persistent:** Understand that meditation is a skill that improves with practice. Be patient with yourself and commit to regular practice, even on days when it feels challenging or you do not notice immediate results.
- **Notice the benefits:** Pay attention to how meditation makes you feel mentally, emotionally, and physically. Notice any changes in your stress levels, mood, and overall well-being as you continue with your practice.

QUESTIONS TO PONDER ON

- How can I incorporate meditation into my daily routine to manage stress more effectively?
- What specific benefits do I hope to gain from establishing a regular meditation practice?
- How can I create a conducive environment for meditation in my home or workspace?
- What guided meditation techniques or resources resonate most with me, and how can I access them regularly?
- How can I stay motivated and committed to my meditation practice, especially during busy or challenging times?

By understanding the intricate relationship between stress and inflammation, and implementing effective stress management techniques like mindfulness and meditation, we can significantly reduce inflammation and improve our overall well-being.

Now, let us dive into the fascinating world of lymphatics and breathing in Chapter 6. Just as we have explored how stress impacts inflammation, we will uncover how optimizing our lymphatic system and harnessing the power of proper breathing techniques can further enhance our health and vitality.

CHAPTER 6
LYMPHATICS AND BREATHING

Move your lymph system. Lymph is like a sewage system that carries all of the toxins out of your body.

- Valentina Zelyaeva

The lymphatic system, often described as the body's drainage network, is a crucial component of our immune system and plays a vital role in maintaining overall health. It consists of a network of vessels, nodes, and organs that work together to circulate lymph fluid throughout the body. This lymph fluid contains white blood cells, known as lymphocytes, which help fight off infections and remove harmful substances from the body.

The lymphatic system plays a critical role in preventing inflammation and promoting overall health by serving as a key component of the body's immune defense and waste removal processes. By circulating lymph fluid throughout the body, the lymphatic system helps to remove toxins, cellular waste, and excess fluids from the tissues, thus, preventing buildup of harmful substances that can trigger inflammation.

Moreover, the lymphatic system functions as a surveillance system for monitoring and capturing pathogens within lymph nodes, such as bacteria and viruses. Here, immune cells called lymphocytes can mount targeted immune responses to neutralize these invaders, hence, preventing infections and reducing the risk of inflammation.

Additionally, the lymphatic system supports tissue repair and regeneration by delivering essential nutrients and immune cells to damaged areas. This helps to accelerate healing and reduce inflammation, therefore, ensures optimal recovery and function.

THE RELATIONSHIP BETWEEN DIAPHRAGMATIC BREATHING AND LYMPHATICS

Diaphragmatic breathing—also known as belly breathing or abdominal breathing—involves the contraction and relaxation of the diaphragm muscle, which separates the chest cavity from the abdominal cavity. It engages the diaphragm more extensively than shallow chest breathing allowing for deeper and more efficient inhalation and exhalation.

When we breathe diaphragmatically, the downward movement of the diaphragm creates negative pressure in the chest cavity, which helps to draw air into the lungs. As the diaphragm contracts, it also massages the thoracic duct—a major lymphatic vessel located near the spine. This gentle massage action promotes the movement of lymphatic fluid through the lymphatic vessels, therefore, facilitating the drainage of toxins, waste products, and excess fluids from the tissues.

Diaphragmatic breathing promotes relaxation and reduces stress by activating the parasympathetic nervous system, often referred to as the "rest and digest" response. This helps to counteract the effects of chronic stress and sympathetic nervous system dominance, which can impair lymphatic function and contribute to inflammation.

Furthermore, diaphragmatic breathing facilitates the flow of lymphatic fluid by stimulating the movement of the lymphatic vessels themselves. The rhythmic expansion and contraction of the thoracic and abdominal cavities during deep breathing act as a gentle massage for the lymphatic vessels that propels lymphatic fluid along its journey toward the lymph nodes and eventually back into the bloodstream.

In addition to its role in promoting optimal lymphatic function, diaphragmatic breathing enhances respiratory efficiency by maximizing the exchange of oxygen and carbon dioxide in the lungs. This supports cellular metabolism and energy production while promoting overall vitality and well-being.

Here are the steps to guide you through diaphragmatic breathing:

- **Find a comfortable position:** Sit or lie down in a comfortable position. You can choose to sit in a chair with your feet flat on the floor or lie down on your back with your knees bent and your feet flat on the bed or floor.
- **Relax your body:** Close your eyes and take a few moments to relax your body. Release any tension you may be holding in your muscles, particularly in your shoulders, neck, and jaw.
- **Place your hands:** You can place one hand on your chest and the other on your abdomen just below your rib cage. This allows you to feel the movement of your diaphragm as you breathe.
- **Inhale slowly through your nose:** Begin by taking a slow, deep breath in through your nose. As you inhale, focus on expanding your abdomen and feeling your hand on your abdomen rise. Allow your chest to remain relatively still.
- **Exhale slowly through your mouth:** After inhaling fully, exhale slowly and steadily through your mouth. As you exhale, gently contract your abdominal muscles to help

expel air from your lungs. Feel your hand on your abdomen lower as you exhale.

- **Repeat:** Continue this slow, deep breathing pattern while focusing on the rise and fall of your abdomen with each breath. Inhale deeply through your nose allowing your abdomen to expand, and exhale slowly through your mouth, gently contracting your abdominal muscles.
- **Practice regularly:** Aim to practice diaphragmatic breathing for at least 5-10 min each day. You can incorporate it into your daily routine by setting aside dedicated time for relaxation and deep breathing exercises.

DRAINAGE TECHNIQUES

To enhance the efficiency of our lymphatic system, we need to focus on techniques that improve drainage, consequently aiding in the removal of toxins and waste products. By incorporating specific drainage techniques into our daily routine, we can support lymphatic health and promote overall well-being.

MANUAL LYMPHATIC DRAINAGE

Manual lymphatic drainage (MLD) is a therapeutic technique aimed at improving lymphatic circulation in the body. It involves gentle, rhythmic massage movements that help stimulate the flow of lymphatic fluid through the lymphatic vessels and nodes. By applying light pressure and specific hand movements along the lymphatic pathways, MLD encourages the removal of excess fluid, toxins, and waste products from the tissues. This technique can be performed by trained professionals or self-administered with proper guidance. MLD is beneficial for reducing swelling, promoting detoxi-fication, and supporting overall lymphatic health.

STEP-BY-STEP GUIDANCE

- Begin by finding a comfortable and quiet space where you can lie down or sit comfortably.
- Start with gentle breathing exercises to help relax your body and mind. Take slow, deep breaths in through your nose, filling your lungs with air, and exhale slowly through your mouth releasing any tension.
- Identify the area of your body where you want to focus the MLD. This could be an area of swelling, discomfort, or where you feel tension.
- Using light pressure, place your fingertips on the skin surface of the chosen area. Make sure your hands are clean and your nails are trimmed to avoid scratching or irritating the skin.
- Gently and rhythmically move your fingertips in a circular or pumping motion following the natural direction of lymphatic flow. Start from the outermost edges of the area and work your way towards the center.
- Repeat the massage strokes several times, gradually increasing the pressure as you feel comfortable. Be mindful not to apply too much pressure, as MLD should be gentle and soothing.
- Continue the massage for about 5–10 min or until you feel a sense of relaxation and relief in the targeted area.
- After completing the MLD session, take a few moments to rest and breathe deeply, and allow your body to fully relax and absorb the benefits of the massage.
- It is essential to drink plenty of water after performing MLD to help flush out toxins and promote lymphatic drainage.

CONTRAST HYDROTHERAPY

Contrast hydrotherapy is a therapeutic technique that involves alternating between hot and cold water applications to specific areas of the body. This method harnesses the contrasting effects of heat and cold to stimulate circulation, reduce inflammation, and promote healing.

Alternating hot and cold water in contrast hydrotherapy stimulates the lymphatic system by dilatating then constricting blood vessels. When exposed to heat, blood vessels allow more blood to flow through them. This increased blood flow brings more oxygen and nutrients to the tissues and encourages the removal of metabolic waste products. Conversely, cold water causes blood vessels to constrict, thus, reducing blood flow to the area. This constriction helps flush out waste materials and toxins from the tissues and promotes the movement of lymphatic fluid.

By alternating between hot and cold water, contrast hydrotherapy creates a pumping action in the lymphatic vessels similar to the effect of muscular contractions during exercise. This pumping action helps propel lymphatic fluid through the vessels, hence, facilitating the drainage of toxins and waste products from the tissues. Additionally, the thermal changes stimulate the activity of immune cells in the lymph nodes, therefore, enhancing the body's ability to fight off infections and reduce inflammation.

QUESTIONS TO PONDER ON

- Have you ever considered the role of your lymphatic system in maintaining your overall health and well-being?
- How often do you practice diaphragmatic breathing or other breathing techniques to support lymphatic function?
- What are some areas of your body where you notice tension or stagnation, and how might improving lymphatic

drainage benefit you?

- Have you tried manual lymphatic drainage techniques before, and if so, what was your experience like?
- Do you incorporate contrast hydrotherapy into your self-care routine, and if not, would you consider giving it a try?
- How do you currently manage inflammation in your body, and could enhancing lymphatic drainage be a beneficial addition to your regimen?
- What challenges do you face in maintaining a healthy lymphatic system, and how might you overcome them?
- Are you aware of any symptoms or signs that may indicate compromised lymphatic function, and if so, how do you address them?

As we journey deeper into understanding inflammation and its impact on our health, it is crucial to explore practical lifestyle changes that can help us effectively manage and reduce inflammation. In the next chapter, we will explore the importance of lifestyle modifications in managing chronic inflammation.

CHAPTER 7

LIFESTYLE CHANGES FOR MANAGING INFLAMMATION

Some people may think you're crazy for giving up certain foods. Some people may think you're even crazier if you work out two or three times a day. Soon enough, they will be asking you how you managed to do it.

- Anonymous

L et us take a moment to reflect on Selena Gomez's journey with her health condition. Despite her immense success in the entertainment industry, Selena Gomez has been open about her battle with lupus—an autoimmune disease that causes chronic inflammation throughout the body. Over the years, she has shared her struggles with managing her health while maintaining a demanding career in the spotlight. Through her advocacy and personal experiences, Selena has highlighted the significance of adopting healthy lifestyle habits to mitigate the effects of inflammation and autoimmune disorders. Her story serves as a poignant reminder of the impact lifestyle changes can have on managing inflammation and promoting overall well-being.

SIGNIFICANCE OF LIFESTYLE MODIFICATIONS

Lifestyle choices exert a profound influence on inflammatory responses serving as key determinants of overall health and well-being. Factors such as diet, physical activity, stress management, sleep patterns, and environmental exposures all contribute to the delicate balance of inflammation within the body. For instance, a diet rich in processed foods, sugars, and unhealthy fats can promote inflammation, while a diet abundant in fruits, vegetables, whole grains, and omega-3 fatty acids can help reduce it. Similarly, regular physical activity has been shown to modulate inflammatory markers and improve immune function, while chronic stress and inadequate sleep can exacerbate inflammation.

By recognizing the pivotal role of lifestyle choices in shaping inflammatory responses, individuals can adopt proactive measures to mitigate inflammation and promote long-term health.

In Chapter 5, we delved into stress management and its crucial role in mitigating inflammation. Next, we will explore in detail the impact of diet, exercise, and sleep on inflammation. Each of these lifestyle factors plays a significant role in either promoting or reducing inflammation in the body.

IMPACT ON AUTOIMMUNE AND OTHER HEALTH CONDITIONS

Lifestyle modifications play a crucial role in managing autoimmune conditions and their symptoms. Let us look at two of the most common autoimmune diseases that can be impacted by lifestyle modifications.

RHEUMATOID ARTHRITIS

Certain dietary patterns, such as the Mediterranean diet rich in fruits, vegetables, whole grains, and healthy fats, have been associated with reduced inflammation and improved outcomes in RA patients. Conversely, diets high in processed foods, refined sugars, and saturated fats may exacerbate inflammation and worsen symptoms.

Regular physical activity is essential for managing RA symptoms, as it helps maintain joint flexibility, strength, and overall function. Low-impact exercises like walking, swimming, and yoga can be particularly beneficial for individuals with RA, as they help reduce inflammation and improve joint mobility without placing excessive stress on the joints.

Chronic stress can exacerbate inflammation and trigger RA flare-ups. Incorporating stress-reduction techniques such as mindfulness meditation, deep breathing exercises, and relaxation therapies can help alleviate stress and promote a sense of well-being, thereby reducing the frequency and severity of RA symptoms.

INFLAMMATORY BOWEL DISEASE

Lifestyle modifications also play a crucial role in managing symptoms and reducing inflammation in individuals with IBD, which includes conditions like Crohn's disease and ulcerative colitis.

Dietary choices can significantly impact IBD symptoms. While specific dietary recommendations may vary depending on individual sensitivities and disease activity, some general principles include avoiding trigger foods such as spicy foods, dairy, caffeine, and alcohol. Instead, focusing on a well-balanced diet rich in fiber, lean proteins, fruits, and vegetables can help support gut health and reduce inflammation.

Regular physical activity is beneficial for individuals with IBD, as it can help improve bowel function, reduce inflammation, and alleviate stress. Low-impact exercises such as walking, cycling, and yoga are generally well-tolerated and can provide numerous health benefits without exacerbating symptoms.

Stress is known to exacerbate IBD symptoms and trigger flare-ups. Therefore, incorporating stress management techniques such as meditation, deep breathing exercises, and relaxation therapies can be beneficial for individuals with IBD. Additionally, seeking support from mental health professionals or joining support groups can provide emotional support and coping strategies to better manage stress.

OVERALL QUALITY OF LIFE ENHANCEMENT

Embracing a holistic approach to lifestyle changes can significantly enhance overall QOL by addressing various aspects of health and well-being. This approach recognizes the interconnectedness of physical, mental, and emotional health, and focuses on optimizing each aspect to promote overall wellness.

One key aspect of enhancing QOL is through proper nutrition. A balanced diet rich in whole foods, fruits, vegetables, lean proteins, and healthy fats provides essential nutrients that support bodily functions, boost immunity, and reduce inflammation. By making mindful food choices and avoiding processed and sugary foods, individuals can maintain energy levels, support gut health, and manage their weight effectively.

Regular physical activity is another crucial component of a holistic lifestyle. Exercise not only strengthens muscles and improves cardiovascular health but also releases endorphins, which are natural mood boosters. Engaging in activities that you enjoy, whether it is walking, dancing, or cycling, can reduce stress, alleviate anxiety, and enhance overall well-being.

In addition to nutrition and exercise, managing stress is paramount for enhancing QOL. Stress-reduction techniques such as meditation, deep breathing exercises, yoga, and mindfulness practices can help calm the mind, promote relaxation, and improve resilience to stressors. By incorporating these practices into their daily routines, individuals can better cope with life's challenges and maintain a sense of balance and inner peace.

Furthermore, fostering social connections and nurturing relationships with loved ones is essential for emotional well-being. Spending quality time with family and friends, engaging in meaningful conversations, and participating in community activities can provide a sense of belonging, support, and fulfillment.

MORGAN FREEMAN

Morgan Freeman, the esteemed actor known for his roles in numerous films including "The Shawshank Redemption" and "Driving Miss Daisy," has been candid about his experience living with fibromyalgia—a chronic pain condition. Freeman has spoken openly about how fibromyalgia affects his daily life and how he manages the symptoms.

Fibromyalgia is characterized by widespread musculoskeletal pain, fatigue, sleep disturbances, and cognitive difficulties. It can be a challenging condition to manage, as its symptoms can fluctuate in intensity and impact various aspects of life.

For Freeman, managing fibromyalgia involves a multifaceted approach that includes lifestyle modifications, stress management techniques, and seeking appropriate medical care. He has highlighted the importance of listening to his body, pacing himself, and prioritizing self-care.

In interviews, Freeman has shared how he incorporates regular exercise, such as swimming and walking, into his routine to help alleviate pain and stiffness associated with fibromyalgia. He also emphasizes the significance of maintaining a healthy diet and staying hydrated to support overall well-being.

Additionally, Freeman practices mindfulness and meditation to reduce stress and promote relaxation, which can help alleviate fibromyalgia symptoms. He advocates for finding activities and practices that bring joy and peace emphasizing the importance of mental and emotional well-being in managing chronic pain.

Despite facing challenges associated with fibromyalgia, Freeman remains resilient and continues to pursue his passion for acting and filmmaking. His openness about his personal experience has helped raise awareness about the condition and has inspired others living with chronic pain to seek support and explore effective management strategies.

QUESTIONS TO PONDER ON

- How do lifestyle choices such as diet, exercise, and stress management influence your overall well-being and QOL?
- Reflect on the impact of your current lifestyle habits on your inflammatory response and autoimmune conditions, if applicable. Are there areas where you can make positive changes?
- Consider the role of stress in exacerbating inflammation and autoimmune symptoms. How can incorporating stress-reduction techniques into your daily routine improve your health outcomes?
- How do you prioritize self-care practices such as adequate sleep, regular physical activity, and mindful eating in managing chronic health conditions and promoting overall wellness?
- Have you noticed any correlations between certain lifestyle factors, such as diet or sleep patterns, and fluctuations in

your symptoms of inflammation or autoimmune disease?

- Reflect on any barriers or challenges you face in implementing lifestyle modifications that support your health goals. How can you overcome these obstacles to foster lasting change?
- What steps can you take to cultivate a holistic approach to lifestyle modifications while considering not only physical health but also mental and emotional well-being?
- How do your personal values and goals align with the lifestyle choices you make to manage inflammation and autoimmune conditions? Are there adjustments you can make to better align with your health priorities?
- Consider the long-term implications of adopting sustainable lifestyle changes for managing chronic health conditions. How do these changes contribute to your overall resilience and QOL?
- Reflect on the role of education and awareness in empowering individuals to make informed decisions about their health and lifestyle. How can you continue to educate yourself and others about the importance of lifestyle modifications in managing inflammation and autoimmune diseases?

In this chapter, we have explored the significant impact of lifestyle modifications on inflammation and autoimmune conditions. By making informed choices about diet, exercise, stress management, sleep, and other lifestyle factors, you can effectively manage your symptoms, enhance your overall QOL, and promote long-term health and well-being.

Next, we will delve into Chapter 8 to uncover the powerful relationship between exercise and inflammation. It is time to incorporate physical exercise into your daily routine.

SHARE YOUR INSIGHTS AND EMPOWER OTHERS

"It is not the strength of the body that counts, but the strength of the spirit."

—*J.R.R. TOLKIEN.*

Take a moment to reflect on the pages of *Inflammation The Silent Fire: Combat Chronic Inflammation With a Science-Backed Approach.* This book wasn't merely a scholarly exploration of inflammation but a companion on your journey to understanding how silent, chronic inflammation can profoundly affect lives—possibly even your own.

Imagine the comfort that your words, derived from personal experience and newfound knowledge, can provide to someone else struggling in silence. Could your story help light the way for them?

This is why I am reaching out to you today with a sincere request:

Would you share your reflections and insights by writing a review?

By detailing your journey and the insights you've gained, you help others in multiple ways:

- Shed light on practical strategies that have worked for you, offering a potential roadmap for others.
- Offer solidarity and understanding to those who feel alone in their health struggles.
- Encourage perseverance by showing others that relief and management are possible.

Each review significantly helps overcome Amazon's algorithms, making it easier for this important book to reach more people who need it. The more visible the book is, the more helpful it can be to someone who feels lost in the face of their health issues.

Your contribution goes beyond just helping to educate others—it's a personal outreach that can profoundly touch others' lives. Here's how you can add your voice:

Please take a brief moment to share your thoughts and review on Amazon at this link, or scan the QR code to be taken to the review page directly:

https://www.amazon.com/review/review-your-purchases/?asin=B0D2B5HCTB

Thank you for considering this request to share your experience. Let's keep the dialogue going and build a community of support and insight against chronic inflammation.

With deepest appreciation,

Dr. Carly Stewart - DPT

P.S. - Your story has immense power. By sharing your experiences, you don't just review a book; you extend a hand of understanding.

You provide not just counsel but also comfort. Let's build a collection of stories that can guide, inspire, and uplift everyone affected by chronic inflammation. Your words are more than a review; they offer hope and a path forward.

CHAPTER 8
PHYSICAL ACTIVITY
AND INFLAMMATION

Take care of your body. It's the only place you have to live.

- Jim Rohn

Paula Abdul—renowned for her dynamic performances as a singer, dancer, and American Idol icon—experienced a setback in 2005 when she was diagnosed with RA. Despite this, she persevered and returned to the stage after treatment. However, in 2015 she encountered new challenges when diagnosed with osteoarthritis after experiencing unusual joint pains during rehearsals. Reflecting on her journey, Abdul expressed relief in understanding the source of her discomfort wishing she had known about the condition earlier.

In a 2020 commercial for Voltaren arthritis gel, Abdul showcased her resilience by dancing alongside a younger version of herself from 1989. Despite her health challenges, Abdul maintains a commitment to regular workouts including low-impact strength exercises and Zumba classes. She emphasizes the importance of movement in maintaining a joyful and healthy life believing that activities like walking—accompanied by music—can be rejuvenating and uplifting (Gerrard, n.d.).

From Abdul's perseverance in returning to the stage to her commitment to regular workouts, her story underscores the profound role of physical activity in maintaining a happy and healthy life despite health challenges. Through the various exercise modalities explored in this chapter, we uncover how movement not only helps manage inflammation but also promotes resilience and vitality.

INFLUENCE OF EXERCISE ON INFLAMMATION

Exercise is not only essential for physical health but also plays a pivotal role in enhancing mental, emotional, and social well-being. Its impact extends beyond just improving physical fitness; regular physical activity has been shown to boost mood, reduce stress and anxiety, and enhance cognitive function. Moreover, engaging in exercise fosters social connections and promotes a sense of belonging and camaraderie, especially when done in group settings or team sports.

In the context of managing chronic inflammation, exercise emerges as a crucial tool. Its multifaceted benefits contribute to mitigating various forms of chronic inflammation by modulating the body's inflammatory responses. Regular exercise helps to optimize immune function, balance hormone levels, and improve circulation—all of which contribute to reducing systemic inflammation. Additionally, exercise promotes the release of endorphins—natural chemicals in the brain that act as pain relievers and mood boosters—further supporting overall well-being.

Firstly, the mechanical stress created when our muscles contract and release during exercise triggers the release of molecules such as cytokines and myokines, which play a role in regulating inflammation. Their pro- or anti-inflammatory effects depend on the intensity and duration of exercise.

While exercise is generally beneficial for health, it is important to acknowledge that certain types or intensities of exercise can indeed trigger inflammation in the body. High-intensity or prolonged exercise sessions, especially when performed without adequate recovery, can lead to a state of overtraining or excessive stress on the body (Cerqueira et al., 2020). In response to this stress, the body may produce higher levels of inflammatory markers leading to acute inflammation. However, this acute inflammatory response is usually followed by a period of reduced inflammation as the body adapts to the stress of exercise.

To mitigate the risk of excessive inflammation from exercise, it is important to engage in a well-regulated exercise routine that includes appropriate warm-up and cool-down periods, adequate rest and recovery between workouts, and gradual progression in intensity and duration. Listening to your body and adjusting your exercise regimen based on how you feel can also help prevent overtraining and excessive inflammation.

On the other hand, chronic exercise, which involves regular and consistent physical activity over time, has been shown to have anti-inflammatory effects. Regular exercise can help to lower levels of pro-inflammatory molecules in the body while increasing the production of anti-inflammatory substances. This chronic reduction in inflammation is believed to contribute to the overall health benefits associated with regular exercise.

TYPES OF EXERCISE

Exercise comes in various forms, each offering unique benefits for our physical and mental well-being. Understanding the different types of exercise is essential for designing a comprehensive fitness regimen that addresses all aspects of health. Each type targets different aspects of fitness and plays a crucial role in promoting overall health and vitality.

AEROBIC EXERCISES

Aerobic exercises, also known as cardiovascular exercises, are activities that increase your heart rate and breathing rate over an extended period of time. These exercises stimulate the circulation of oxygen-rich blood throughout the body, supporting the efficient functioning of various organs and systems, including the immune system. Aerobic exercise can help manage inflammation by reducing levels of pro-inflammatory markers and promoting the release of anti-inflammatory substances in the body.

Here are five practical aerobic exercises along with steps that you can follow.

BRISK WALKING

- Find a safe and comfortable place to walk, such as a park or neighborhood sidewalk.
- Start with a gentle warm-up by walking at a slower pace for 5–10 min.
- Gradually increase your pace to a brisk walk until you can still hold a conversation but feel slightly breathless.
- Aim for a duration of at least 30 min gradually increasing to 60 min or more as your fitness improves.
- Cool down by walking at a slower pace for 5–10 min followed by gentle stretching.

CYCLING

- Choose a stationary bike or ride outdoors on a safe route.

- Begin with a light warm-up pedaling at a comfortable pace for 5–10 min.
- Increase your pedaling intensity to a moderate or vigorous level maintaining a steady pace.
- Aim for a duration of 20–60 min depending on your fitness level and goals.
- Cool down by pedaling at a slower pace for 5–10 min then stretching your lower body muscles.

SWIMMING

- Find a swimming pool or open water area with lifeguards present.
- Start with a few laps of easy swimming to warm up your muscles and joints.
- Progress to swimming continuous laps at a moderate to vigorous intensity using various strokes like freestyle, backstroke, breaststroke, or butterfly.
- Aim for a duration of 20–45 min adjusting based on your swimming ability and fitness level.
- Cool down by swimming at an easy pace for a few laps followed by gentle stretching in the water or on the pool deck.

DANCING

- Choose your favorite style of dance such as salsa, hip-hop, or Zumba.
- Begin with a dynamic warm-up including movements like marching, arm circles, and gentle stretches.
- Dance to upbeat music, focusing on moving your entire body and increasing your heart rate.

- Aim for a duration of 30–60 min while adjusting the intensity based on the tempo of the music and your comfort level.
- Cool down with slower dance movements and gentle stretching to relax your muscles.

JUMP ROPE

- Find a flat, non-slip surface with enough space to jump rope safely.
- Start with a light warm-up, including dynamic stretches for your calves, thighs, and shoulders.
- Begin jumping rope at a moderate pace, focusing on maintaining good form and rhythm.
- Aim for a duration of 10-20 minutes, gradually increasing as your endurance improves.
- Cool down by slowing your pace and performing static stretches for your lower body muscles.

To optimize the inflammatory response, aim for aerobic exercises that elevate your heart rate to a moderate-to-vigorous intensity level. This typically means exercising at an intensity where you can still talk but would find it challenging to sing. Aim for at least 150 min of moderate-intensity aerobic exercise or 75 min of vigorous-intensity aerobic exercise per week spread out over several sessions. Additionally, incorporating both continuous and interval training can provide added benefits for managing inflammation and improving overall cardiovascular health.

ANAEROBIC EXERCISES

Anaerobic exercises are high-intensity activities that involve short bursts of energy without relying on oxygen for fuel. These exercises primarily target muscle strength, power, and endurance, subsequently contributing to overall fitness and health. In the context of inflammation management, anaerobic exercise plays a crucial role in promoting anti-inflammatory effects by stimulating muscle growth, improving insulin sensitivity, and enhancing metabolic function.

WEIGHTLIFTING

Resistance training using free weights or weight machines targets specific muscle groups leading to increased muscle mass and strength. Compound exercises like squats, deadlifts, dumbbell rolls and bench presses engage multiple muscle groups simultaneously, hence, providing a comprehensive workout.

Squats

- Stand with your feet shoulder-width apart, toes slightly turned out.
- Engage your core and keep your chest up as you lower your body by bending your knees and hips.
- Lower yourself down as if sitting back into a chair keeping your knees in line with your toes.
- Descend until your thighs are parallel to the ground or slightly below, ensuring your knees do not go past your toes.
- Drive through your heels to return to the starting position and squeeze your glutes at the top.
- Repeat for the desired number of repetitions.

Deadlifts

- Stand with your feet hip-width apart, toes pointing forward, and a barbell on the ground in front of you.
- Bend at your hips and knees to lower your torso keeping your back straight and chest up.

- Grip the barbell with both hands slightly wider than shoulder-width apart, palms facing you or mixed grip.
- Engage your core, push through your heels, and lift the barbell by extending your hips and knees simultaneously.
- Keep the barbell close to your body as you stand up straight while maintaining a neutral spine.
- Slowly lower the barbell back to the ground by hinging at your hips and bending your knees.
- Repeat for the desired number of repetitions.

Bench Press

- Lie flat on a bench with your feet planted firmly on the ground shoulder-width apart.
- Grip the barbell slightly wider than shoulder-width apart (palms facing away from you).
- Lower the barbell to your chest by bending your elbows, keeping them close to your body at a 45° angle.
- Pause briefly when the barbell touches your chest.
- Push the barbell back up to the starting position by extending your elbows and squeezing your chest muscles.
- Keep your back flat and avoid arching excessively.
- Repeat for the desired number of repetitions.

Dumbbell Rows

- Start by placing one knee and the same-side hand on a flat bench keeping your back flat and parallel to the ground.
- Hold a dumbbell in the opposite hand with your arm extended towards the floor—palm facing inward.
- Keep your core engaged as you pull the dumbbell up towards your hip by bending your elbow while keeping it close to your body.

- Squeeze your shoulder blade at the top of the movement, then lower the dumbbell back down with control.
- Repeat for the desired number of repetitions, then switch sides and perform the same movement with the other arm.

These exercises target different muscle groups and are effective for building strength and muscle mass, which can help support your joints and reduce inflammation. Start with a weight that challenges you but allows you to maintain proper form, and gradually increase the resistance as you get stronger. As always, prioritize safety and proper technique to prevent injury.

BODYWEIGHT EXERCISES

Exercises such as push-ups, pull-ups, and lunges use your body weight as resistance to build strength and endurance. These exercises can be modified to suit different fitness levels and can be performed anywhere without the need for specialized equipment.

Push-Ups

- Start in a plank position with your hands slightly wider than shoulder-width apart and your body forming a straight line from head to heels.
- Engage your core and lower your body towards the ground by bending your elbows keeping them close to your sides.
- Lower yourself until your chest nearly touches the ground, then push through your palms to return to the starting position.
- Keep your body straight throughout the movement while avoiding sagging or arching your back.
- Repeat for the desired number of repetitions.

Pull-Ups

- Hang from a pull-up bar with an overhand grip, hands slightly wider than shoulder-width apart.
- Engage your core and pull yourself up towards the bar by bending your elbows and squeezing your shoulder blades together.
- Continue pulling until your chin clears the bar, then lower yourself back down with control.
- Keep your movements slow and controlled and avoid swinging or using momentum.
- Repeat for the desired number of repetitions.

Lunges

- Start standing with your feet hip-width apart and your hands on your hips or by your sides.
- Take a step forward with one foot, lowering your body until both knees are bent at a 90° angle.
- Keep your front knee aligned with your ankle and your back knee hovering just above the ground.
- Push through your front heel to return to the starting position, then repeat on the other side.
- Alternate legs with each repetition while ensuring smooth and controlled movements.
- Repeat for the desired number of repetitions on each leg.

Bodyweight Squats

- Begin by standing with your feet shoulder-width apart and toes pointed slightly outward.
- Engage your core and lower your body by bending your knees and pushing your hips back as if sitting into an imaginary chair.
- Keep your chest up and your back straight throughout the movement, as your knees track in line with your toes.

- Lower yourself until your thighs are parallel to the ground or as far down as comfortable.
- Push through your heels to return to the starting position while fully extending your hips and knees.
- Repeat for the desired number of repetitions while maintaining control and proper form.

Planks

- Start in a plank position with your elbows directly beneath your shoulders and your body forming a straight line from head to heels.
- Engage your core muscles and hold this position while avoiding sagging or arching your back.
- Keep your neck in line with your spine and your gaze directed towards the floor.
- Hold the plank for a specified amount of time aiming to maintain proper form throughout.
- Focus on breathing steadily and evenly as you hold the position.
- To modify, you can perform the plank on your knees or elevate your hands on an elevated surface.
- Gradually increase the duration of your plank hold as your core strength improves.

These bodyweight exercises target multiple muscle groups and can be incorporated into your workout routine to improve strength, stability, and overall fitness. As with any exercise program, it is essential to perform movements in proper form to prevent injury and maximize benefits.

PLYOMETRIC EXERCISES

Plyometric exercises, such as box jumps, jump squats, burpees, mountain climbers and jump lunges, involve explosive movements that improve muscle power and coordination. These exercises enhance neuromuscular function and promote muscle activation, hence, aid in inflammation management.

Box Jumps

- Start by standing in front of a sturdy box or platform with your feet shoulder-width apart.
- Lower yourself into a quarter squat position swinging your arms back for momentum.
- Explosively jump onto the box, extending your hips, knees, and ankles fully.
- Land softly on the box while absorbing the impact by bending your knees.
- Step down carefully from the box and repeat for the desired number of repetitions.

Jump Squats

- Begin by standing with your feet shoulder-width apart and arms at your sides.
- Lower into a squat position keeping your chest up and your weight on your heels.
- Explosively jump into the air while extending your hips and knees fully.
- As you jump, swing your arms overhead for momentum.
- Land softly bending your knees to absorb the impact, and immediately lower into the next squat.
- Repeat the movement for the desired number of repetitions while maintaining a controlled pace.

Burpees

- Start in a standing position with your feet shoulder-width apart.
- Lower into a squat position and place your hands on the ground in front of you.
- Kick your feet back into a plank position keeping your body straight from head to heels.
- Perform a push-up by bending your elbows and lowering your chest towards the ground.
- Push through your palms to return to the plank position.
- Jump your feet back towards your hands and explosively jump into the air, reaching your arms overhead.
- Land softly and immediately lower back into the squat position to begin the next repetition.
- Repeat the exercise for the desired number of repetitions maintaining proper form throughout.

Mountain Climbers

- Start in a plank position with your hands directly under your shoulders and your body forming a straight line from head to heels.
- Engage your core muscles and lift your right foot off the ground bringing your right knee towards your chest.
- Quickly switch legs bringing your right foot back and your left knee towards your chest.
- Continue alternating legs in a running motion moving as quickly as possible while maintaining proper plank form.
- Perform the exercise for the desired duration or number of repetitions keeping your movements controlled and steady.

Jump Lunges

- Begin in a lunge position with your right leg forward, knee bent at a 90° angle, and your left leg extended behind you.
- Lower into a lunge ensuring your front knee stays aligned with your ankle and your back knee hovers just above the ground.
- Explosively jump into the air switching the position of your legs mid-air so that your left leg is now forward and your right leg is extended behind you.
- Land softly, immediately lowering into a lunge position on the opposite side.
- Continue alternating legs with each jump maintaining a steady pace and proper form throughout.
- Perform the exercise for the desired number of repetitions or duration focusing on engaging your leg muscles and maintaining balance.

These plyometric exercises are effective for improving explosive power, coordination, and muscle activation. Incorporate them into your workout routine gradually and ensure proper form to minimize the risk of injury and maximize benefits.

HIGH-INTENSITY INTERVAL TRAINING

High-intensity interval training (HIIT) workouts involve alternating between short bursts of intense exercise and brief periods of rest or low-intensity activity. This form of exercise boosts cardiovascular fitness, enhances metabolic rate, and promotes fat loss—all of which contribute to reducing inflammation.

SPRINTING

Short, intense sprints challenge your muscles and cardiovascular system, improving speed, power, and agility. Sprinting also stimulates the release of growth hormone and testosterone, which have anti-inflammatory properties.

FLEXIBILITY EXERCISES

Flexibility exercises play a crucial role in inflammation management by promoting muscle relaxation, improving joint mobility, and reducing tension in the body. Practices such as yoga and stretching help alleviate stiffness and soreness, therefore, enhancing overall flexibility and range of motion. The increase of blood flow by gently lengthening and stretching the muscles and connective tissues aids in the reduction of metabolic waste products and inflammation.

Additionally, these exercises can help alleviate stress and promote relaxation, further contributing to inflammation reduction. Regular participation in flexibility exercises can improve overall physical function, prevent injury, and support a healthy inflammatory response in the body.

You can start with these five yoga poses.

CHILD'S POSE (BALASANA)

- Start on your hands and knees with your wrists directly under your shoulders and your knees hip-width apart.
- Sit back on your heels and lower your torso down toward the floor extending your arms in front of you.
- Rest your forehead on the mat and relax your neck and shoulders.
- Hold the pose for 30 s to 1 min while focusing on deep breathing.

DOWNWARD-FACING DOG (ADHO MUKHA SVANASANA)

- Begin on your hands and knees with your wrists slightly in front of your shoulders and your knees hip-width apart.
- Lift your hips up and back as you straighten your arms and legs to form an inverted V shape.
- Press your palms into the mat and lengthen your spine reaching your heels toward the floor.
- Hold the pose for 30 s to 1 min focusing on elongating your spine and relaxing your neck.

STANDING FORWARD FOLD (UTTANASANA)

- Stand with your feet hip-width apart and hinge forward at your hips, bending your knees slightly if necessary.
- Let your upper body hang forward allowing your head and arms to dangle toward the floor.
- Hold onto opposite elbows with your hands or let your hands rest on the floor or grab onto your ankles.
- Relax your neck and shoulders, and breathe deeply into your hamstrings and lower back.
- Hold the pose for 30 s to 1 min, gently swaying from side to side if it feels comfortable.

SEATED FORWARD BEND (PASCHIMOTTANASANA)

- Sit on the floor with your legs extended in front of you and your feet flexed toward you.
- Inhale to lengthen your spine, then exhale to hinge forward at your hips, reaching for your shins, ankles, or feet.
- Keep your back straight as you fold forward leading with your chest and keeping your neck in line with your spine.
- Hold onto your legs or feet and relax your head and neck.

- Hold the pose for 30 s to 1 min breathing deeply into your lower back and hamstrings.

CAT-COW STRETCH (MARJARYASANA-BITILASANA)

- Begin on your hands and knees with your wrists directly under your shoulders and your knees hip-width apart.
- Inhale as you arch your back dropping your belly toward the floor and lifting your tailbone and gaze toward the ceiling (Cow Pose).
- Exhale as you round your spine, tuck your chin toward your chest, and draw your navel toward your spine (Cat Pose).
- Continue flowing between Cat and Cow Poses with each inhale and exhale moving at your own pace for 5-10 rounds.

Practice these yoga poses or stretches regularly to improve flexibility, reduce tension, and promote relaxation in your body and mind.

MANAGING CHRONIC INFLAMMATION THROUGH PHYSICAL ACTIVITY

Emphasizing enjoyment and sustainability in maintaining a regular exercise practice is crucial for long-term success. When you genuinely enjoy the physical activities you engage in, you are more likely to stick with them over time. Look for activities that bring you joy, whether it is dancing, hiking, playing sports, or practicing yoga. By incorporating activities you love into your exercise routine, you will feel motivated to stay active and look forward to your workouts.

Additionally, sustainability is key to maintaining consistency in your exercise practice. Choose activities that fit seamlessly into your lifestyle and schedule, thus, alleviate prioritizing regular physical activity. Whether it is finding time for a morning walk, joining a fitness class with friends, or incorporating exercise breaks into your workday, aim for manageable and sustainable habits that you can maintain in the long run.

Combining exercise with other lifestyle changes can have synergistic effects, thereby enhancing the overall management of inflammation. When exercise is paired with dietary adjustments, stress management techniques, and improved sleep hygiene, it creates a holistic approach that addresses various aspects of health and well-being.

Exercise complements dietary adjustments by promoting weight management, improving insulin sensitivity, and enhancing metabolic function. Regular physical activity helps regulate blood sugar levels, which can reduce inflammation associated with conditions like diabetes and metabolic syndrome. Additionally, exercise can increase nutrient absorption and support a healthy gut microbiome, further contributing to inflammation reduction.

Furthermore, exercise is an effective tool for stress management, as it helps release endorphins—the body's natural stress relievers. By incorporating physical activity into your daily routine, you can alleviate stress and tension, which in turn reduces the production of stress hormones like cortisol that contribute to inflammation. Engaging in activities like yoga or tai chi, which combine movement with mindfulness practices, can be particularly beneficial for stress reduction and inflammation management.

Additionally, exercise plays a crucial role in promoting restful sleep and improving sleep quality. Regular physical activity helps regulate circadian rhythms and promotes relaxation, thus, enables falling and staying asleep throughout the night. By incorporating exercise into your daily routine, you can establish healthy sleep patterns that support optimal recovery and inflammation management.

CREATING AN EXERCISE ROUTINE FOR INFLAMMATION MANAGEMENT

When creating an exercise routine for inflammation management, it is important to recognize that the challenge may not always lie in the intensity of the exercises, but rather in the consistency of your efforts. Consistency is key when it comes to reaping the benefits of physical activity for inflammation reduction.

Instead of focusing solely on high-intensity workouts or pushing yourself to the limit every time you exercise, prioritize consistency by incorporating regular, moderate-intensity activities into your routine. This could include activities like brisk walking, swimming, cycling, or gentle yoga sessions.

By committing to a consistent exercise schedule, you can gradually build strength, endurance, and resilience over time without placing excessive strain on your body. Consistency allows you to establish healthy habits and maintain a sustainable approach to physical activity, which is essential for long-term inflammation management.

- **Set realistic goals:** Begin by setting achievable goals based on your current fitness level, health status, and personal preferences. Whether you aim for a certain quantity of workouts or intensity, setting realistic goals will help you stay motivated and track your progress.
- **Choose activities you enjoy:** Select physical activities that you genuinely enjoy and look forward to doing. Whether it is brisk walking, swimming, cycling, or dancing, finding activities that bring you joy will make it easier to stick to your exercise routine in the long run.
- **Incorporate variety:** Include a variety of exercises in your routine to target different muscle groups and prevent boredom. Mix cardiovascular and strength training activities like walking or jogging and weightlifting or

bodyweight workouts, respectively. Adding flexibility exercises like yoga or stretching can also improve mobility and reduce muscle tension.

- **Gradually increase intensity:** Start with low to moderate-intensity workouts and gradually increase the intensity as your fitness level improves. Listen to your body and avoid pushing yourself too hard, especially if you are new to exercise or have existing health conditions. Gradual progression allows your body to adapt safely and reduces the risk of injury.
- **Prioritize consistency:** Consistency is key when it comes to reaping the benefits of exercise for inflammation management. Aim for regular, consistent workouts rather than sporadic, intense sessions. Even shorter bouts of exercise spread throughout the day can be effective in improving overall health and reducing inflammation.
- **Listen to your body:** Pay attention to how your body responds to exercise and adjust your routine accordingly. If you experience pain, fatigue, or other discomfort during or after exercise, modify your activities or seek guidance from a healthcare professional. It is important to find a balance between challenging yourself and respecting your body's limits.
- **Include rest and recovery:** Incorporate rest days into your exercise routine to allow your body time to recover and repair. Rest is essential for preventing overtraining and reducing the risk of injury. Use rest days to engage in gentle activities like walking, stretching, or yoga, and prioritize quality sleep to support recovery.

QUESTIONS TO PONDER ON

- How can I prioritize consistency in my exercise routine to better manage inflammation over time?

- What types of physical activities do I enjoy and feel motivated to engage in regularly?
- How can I adjust my exercise routine to accommodate fluctuations in energy levels or physical discomfort?
- What role do rest and recovery play in optimizing the effectiveness of my exercise regimen for inflammation management?
- How can I cultivate a positive mindset towards physical activity to make it an enjoyable and sustainable part of my lifestyle?

In our journey to explore lifestyle modifications for managing inflammation, we now turn our attention to the crucial role of sleep. Just as exercise, diet, and stress management influence inflammation, sleep also plays a significant part in regulating our body's inflammatory responses.

CHAPTER 9
SLEEP AND INFLAMMATION

In whatever disease sleep is laborious, it is a deadly symptom; but if sleep does good, it is not deadly.

- Hippocrates

We are all familiar with LeBron James, are we not? The iconic professional basketball player is known for his exceptional skills on the court. LeBron credits a significant portion of his athletic prowess to the quality of his sleep regimen. With a steadfast dedication to obtaining 8–10 h of rest each night, he emphasizes how this practice sharpens his focus and enhances his performance during games. LeBron's emphasis on the importance of adequate sleep underscores its critical role in optimizing physical and mental capabilities as well as overall health and wellness.

RELATIONSHIP BETWEEN SLEEP QUALITY, CIRCADIAN RHYTHMS, AND INFLAMMATION

Good-quality sleep is like giving your body proper maintenance to run smoothly. But when your sleep quality is poor, it is like neglecting to take care of that machine. Without proper rest, your body cannot repair itself effectively, and things start to go awry.

But when you do not get enough sleep, your body's inflammatory response can go haywire. It is like sending out too many soldiers for a small skirmish; things get chaotic and innocent bystanders—your healthy cells—get caught in the crossfire. This leads to inflammation running rampant throughout your body causing all sorts of problems like swelling, pain, and even chronic diseases.

Poor sleep quality disrupts the delicate balance of your body's inflammatory response leading to increased inflammation and potential health issues. It is essential to prioritize good sleep habits to keep inflammation in check and maintain overall well-being.

CIRCADIAN RHYTHMS AND INFLAMMATION

Think of your body as having its own built-in clock following the circadian rhythm—a natural alarm system that tells you when it is time to wake up or wind down for sleep. Now, just like how you set your alarm to wake you up at the same time every day, your body follows a similar schedule based on its circadian rhythm.

Now, here's where it gets interesting: your circadian rhythm does not just regulate your sleep-wake cycle; it also influences other bodily functions, including inflammation. You see, your body is designed to be in sync with the natural cycles of day and night. When you disrupt this rhythm by staying up late or waking up irregularly, it is like throwing a wrench into the gears of your body's internal clock.

When your circadian rhythm is out of whack, it can throw off the timing of important processes in your body, including inflammation regulation. Your body might start producing inflammatory molecules at the wrong times leading to increased inflammation and potential health issues.

Quality sleep plays a crucial role in managing chronic inflammation in several ways:

- **Regulating inflammatory pathways:** During sleep, the body undergoes various repair and restoration processes, including the regulation of inflammatory pathways. Adequate sleep helps balance the production of pro- and anti-inflammatory cytokines, which are key molecules involved in the body's immune response. By promoting this balance, quality sleep helps prevent excessive inflammation.
- **Supporting immune function:** Sleep is essential for maintaining a healthy immune system. Chronic sleep deprivation can weaken immune function making the body more susceptible to infections and inflammatory conditions. By ensuring sufficient sleep, the body can better defend against pathogens and regulate inflammatory responses.
- **Reducing stress levels:** Poor sleep can increase stress hormone levels such as cortisol in the body. Elevated cortisol levels contribute to systemic inflammation and can exacerbate chronic inflammatory conditions. Conversely, adequate sleep helps regulate cortisol levels, conversely reducing stress and inflammation.
- **Improving tissue repair:** Sleep is crucial for tissue repair and regeneration. During sleep, the body repairs damaged tissues and cells including those affected by inflammation. By promoting efficient tissue repair, quality sleep helps

mitigate the inflammatory damage caused by various conditions.

- **Enhancing metabolic health:** Chronic sleep deprivation is associated with metabolic disturbances such as insulin resistance and obesity, which can contribute to systemic inflammation. Quality sleep can support metabolic health, by reducing inflammation.

TIPS FOR IMPROVING SLEEP HYGIENE AND HABITS

Ensuring a good night's sleep is essential for our overall health and well-being. Sleep hygiene refers to the habits and practices that promote quality sleep and optimize our restorative rest. From creating a comfortable sleep environment to adopting healthy bedtime routines, improving sleep hygiene can have a profound impact on our ability to fall and stay asleep, and wake up feeling refreshed.

CREATING A SLEEP-INDUCING ENVIRONMENT

Optimizing your bedroom environment can significantly improve your sleep quality and help minimize inflammation. Here are some tips for creating a sleep-friendly space:

- **Control temperature:** Keep your bedroom cool and comfortable. The optimal temperature for sleep is typically between 60 and 67 °F (15.5 to 19.5 °C). Adjust your thermostat or use fans or air conditioning to maintain a cool temperature conducive to sleep.
- **Manage lighting:** Minimize exposure to bright lights in the evening hours, especially blue light from electronic devices. as it can disrupt your body's natural sleep-wake cycle by suppressing the production of melatonin—a hormone that

regulates sleep. Use blackout curtains or sleep masks to block out external light sources and create a dark sleep environment.

- **Reduce noise:** Eliminate or reduce disruptive noises that may disturb your sleep. Consider using earplugs or a white noise machine to mask unwanted sounds such as traffic or household noise. Alternatively, you can use soothing sounds like nature sounds or calming music to promote relaxation and mask background noise.

- **Comfortable bedding:** Invest in a comfortable mattress and pillows that provide adequate support for your body. Choose bedding materials that are breathable and conducive to temperature regulation, such as cotton or bamboo sheets. Ensure your sleep surface is comfortable and free of lumps or sagging that may disrupt sleep.

- **Declutter and organize:** Keep your bedroom clean, clutter-free, and organized to create a calming and relaxing environment. Clutter can contribute to stress and anxiety, which may interfere with sleep quality. Create a serene and inviting space that promotes relaxation and restorative sleep.

ESTABLISHING CONSISTENT SLEEP PATTERNS

Maintaining consistent sleep and wake times is crucial for syncing your circadian rhythm, which regulates various physiological processes including sleep-wake cycles and inflammation. Here are some tips to help you establish and maintain consistent sleep patterns:

- **Set a regular sleep schedule:** Aim to go to bed and wake up at the same time every day, even on weekends. Consistency reinforces your body's internal clock and promotes better sleep quality over time.

- **Create a bedtime routine:** Develop a relaxing pre-sleep routine to signal to your body that it is time to wind down. Activities like reading, taking a warm bath, or practicing relaxation techniques can help prepare your mind and body for sleep.
- **Limit exposure to screens:** Minimize exposure to electronic devices before bedtime, such as smartphones, tablets, and computers. The blue light emitted by screens can suppress melatonin production and disrupt your sleep-wake cycle. Consider implementing a "screen curfew" at least an hour before bedtime.
- **Avoid napping late in the day:** While short naps can be beneficial for some people, avoid napping too close to bedtime as it can interfere with your ability to fall asleep at night. If you need to nap, aim for early to mid-afternoon and limit it to 20-30 min.

SCREEN TIME AND SLEEP

Electronic devices such as smartphones, tablets, computers, and televisions have become ubiquitous in modern society, but their excessive use—particularly before bedtime—can have detrimental effects on sleep quality and disrupt circadian rhythms.

Screens emit blue light, which can suppress the production of melatonin, the hormone that regulates sleep-wake cycles. Exposure to blue light in the evening can trick your brain into thinking it is still daytime, making it harder to fall asleep and stay asleep.

Engaging with screens, whether it is scrolling through social media, watching videos, or playing games, can be mentally stimulating and keep your mind alert when it should be winding down for sleep. This heightened arousal can delay the onset of sleep and reduce sleep quality.

Using screens late into the night can disrupt your body's internal clock, or circadian rhythm, which regulates various physiological processes including sleep-wake cycles. Irregular sleep-wake patterns can lead to insomnia, daytime sleepiness, and overall sleep disturbances.

To minimize the negative impact of screen time on sleep hygiene, consider implementing the following tips:

- **Establish a screen curfew:** Set a specific time in the evening when you will stop using electronic devices and begin winding down for bed. Aim to disconnect from screens at least an hour before bedtime to allow your brain to transition into sleep mode.
- **Use night Mode or blue light filters:** Many electronic devices offer a night mode or blue light filter feature that reduces the amount of blue light emitted by the screen. Enable these settings in the evening to minimize the impact on melatonin production and promote better sleep.
- **Create a tech-free bedroom:** Keep electronic devices out of the bedroom or at least out of arm's reach while you are winding down for bed. Designate your bedroom as a screen-free zone to promote relaxation and signal to your brain that it's time to sleep.
- **Engage in relaxing activities:** Replace screen time with calming activities that promote relaxation and prepare your mind and body for sleep. Consider reading a book, practicing gentle stretching or yoga, or listening to soothing music or white noise.
- **Establish a bedtime routine:** Develop a consistent bedtime routine that does not involve screens. Engage in relaxing activities that signal to your body that it is time to sleep such as taking a warm bath, practicing deep breathing exercises, or journaling.

LIMITING STIMULANTS AND HEAVY MEALS BEFORE BED

Your dietary choices, especially in the hours leading up to bedtime, can significantly impact your sleep quality and inflammation levels.

Substances like caffeine, nicotine, and certain medications can act as stimulants, increasing alertness and arousal and making it difficult to fall asleep. Consuming stimulants too close to bedtime can delay the onset of sleep and reduce overall sleep quality. Additionally, stimulants can disrupt the natural sleep cycle, leading to fragmented or shallow sleep, which may not provide the same restorative benefits as deep, uninterrupted sleep.

Eating large or heavy meals close to bedtime can also negatively impact sleep quality. Digesting a heavy meal requires energy and metabolic activity, which can interfere with the body's ability to transition into a relaxed state conducive to sleep. Additionally, lying down after a heavy meal can exacerbate symptoms of acid reflux or indigestion, further disrupting sleep and increasing discomfort.

To optimize your sleep quality and inflammation management, consider the following recommendations:

- **Avoid caffeine and nicotine:** Limit your consumption of caffeinated beverages such as coffee, tea, and soda, especially in the afternoon and evening hours. Similarly, avoid using nicotine-containing products like cigarettes or electronic cigarettes close to bedtime, as nicotine is a stimulant that can interfere with sleep onset and quality.
- **Monitor medication use:** Be mindful of any medications you take that may contain stimulants or have stimulating effects. Consult with your healthcare provider about the timing of medication administration to minimize its impact on sleep.
- **Opt for lighter meals:** Instead of heavy or rich meals, choose lighter, easily digestible options for your evening

meal. Focus on incorporating lean proteins, whole grains, fruits, and vegetables into your dinner to provide essential nutrients without overburdening your digestive system.

- **Limit spicy or acidic Foods:** Spicy or acidic foods can exacerbate symptoms of acid reflux or heartburn, which can disrupt sleep and cause discomfort. Avoid consuming these types of foods close to bedtime to minimize the risk of digestive issues interfering with your sleep.

- **Allow time for digestion:** Aim to finish eating at least 2–3 h before bedtime to allow ample time for digestion before lying down. If you experience hunger before bed, opt for a light snack that will not overload your digestive system or cause discomfort.

PHYSICAL ACTIVITY AND MINDFUL RELAXATION TECHNIQUES

Combining physical exercise with mindful relaxation techniques can significantly improve sleep quality by promoting relaxation, reducing stress, and regulating circadian rhythms. We have already explored the individual benefits of physical exercise and mindful meditation in previous chapters, and now we have to establish that combining these practices can enhance sleep quality even further.

Engaging in regular physical activity, such as aerobic exercises, strength training, or yoga, helps release tension from the body and promote feelings of relaxation. Exercise triggers the release of endorphins, which are natural mood lifters, and reduces levels of stress hormones like cortisol. Incorporating physical exercise into your daily routine can tire your body in a healthy way, hence, facilitating falling and staying asleep throughout the night.

Mindfulness meditation, deep breathing exercises, and progressive muscle relaxation are effective techniques for calming the mind and body before bedtime. These practices help alleviate anxiety, quiet racing thoughts, and promote a sense of inner peace conducive to sleep. By practicing mindfulness regularly, you can train your mind to let go of worries and distractions, thereby allowing you to relax more deeply and fall asleep more easily.

PREPARING FOR RESTFUL SLEEP

As we conclude this chapter, I encourage you to try a simple relaxation exercise to help prepare your mind and body for restful sleep:

- Find a comfortable position in bed lying on your back with your arms resting gently by your sides.
- Close your eyes and take a few slow, deep breaths inhaling deeply through your nose and exhaling fully through your mouth.
- Begin to tense and release each muscle group in your body starting with your toes and working your way up to your head. As you tense each muscle group, hold the tension for a few seconds, then release and allow the muscles to relax completely.
- Continue this process, moving through your feet, calves, thighs, abdomen, chest, arms, and finally, your face and neck. Pay attention to any areas of tension or discomfort, and consciously release the tension with each exhale.
- Once you have relaxed all the muscles in your body, focus on your breath. Take slow, deep breaths in and out allowing each breath to deepen your state of relaxation.
- If your mind starts to wander or you notice any distracting thoughts, gently bring your attention back to your breath and the sensation of relaxation in your body.
- Remain in this relaxed state for as long as you like allowing yourself to drift off into a peaceful and rejuvenating sleep.

Continuing our journey through lifestyle modifications for managing inflammation, let us delve into Chapter 10.

THE ROLE OF DIET IN MANAGING INFLAMMATION

Joint pain, bloating, and foggy thoughts are not imagined symptoms; they're the result of an improper diet. Make eliminations. Start with wheat, then dairy, then sugar. These are the most inflammatory foods.

- Nancy S. Mure

T om Brady, the renowned quarterback for the New England Patriots, follows a strict, plant-based diet carefully curated to prioritize foods believed to combat inflammation. His personal chef, Allen Campbell, reveals the key components of Brady's diet that exclude certain foods deemed pro-inflammatory. These exclusions encompass a wide range of items including white sugar, white flour, monosodium glutamate (MSG), and canola oil, which can potentially transform into trans fats—unsaturated fatty acids originating from the meat and milk of ruminant animals. Instead, Campbell opts for raw olive oil sparingly and primarily cooks with coconut oil. To season dishes, he relies on Himalayan pink salt for its lower sodium content compared to iodized salt. Nightshade vegetables such as tomatoes, peppers, mushrooms, and eggplants are notably absent from Brady's diet due to their perceived inflammatory properties. Although tomatoes may occasionally make an appearance, they are consumed sparingly. Additionally, Brady abstains from coffee, caffeine, fungus, and dairy products as part of his inflammation-reducing regimen (Belluz, 2016).

The role of diet in managing inflammation emphasizes the crucial distinction between selecting foods solely for taste and choosing those that serve as fuel for our bodies, hence, aid in the battle against inflammation.

IMPORTANCE OF A BALANCED, NUTRIENT-RICH DIET

A balanced, nutrient-rich diet is essential for managing inflammation and promoting overall well-being. This type of diet provides the body with the necessary nutrients to support a healthy inflammatory response and maintain optimal function of various bodily systems. Essential nutrients including vitamins, minerals, and other micronutrients play key roles in regulating inflammation and supporting overall health.

Vitamins: Certain vitamins play crucial roles in modulating inflammation. For example, vitamin C is a powerful antioxidant that scavenges free radicals and reduces oxidative stress, while vitamin D helps regulate the immune system and has anti-inflammatory effects. Vitamin E also acts as an antioxidant and helps protect cell membranes from damage by free radicals. Additionally, vitamins B6 and B12 play roles in immune function and may help reduce inflammation.

Minerals: Minerals such as magnesium, zinc, and selenium are important for maintaining a healthy inflammatory response. Magnesium helps regulate muscle and nerve function, blood sugar levels, and blood pressure, while zinc supports immune function and wound healing. Selenium acts as an antioxidant and may help reduce inflammation by neutralizing free radicals.

Omega-3 fatty acids: Omega-3 fatty acids, found in fatty fish like salmon, mackerel, and sardines, as well as in flaxseeds, chia seeds, and walnuts, are well-known for their anti-inflammatory properties. These essential fatty acids help reduce inflammation by inhibiting the production of pro-inflammatory molecules called cytokines and prostaglandins.

Antioxidants: Antioxidants are compounds that help neutralize free radicals and reduce oxidative stress, thereby reducing inflammation. Examples include beta-carotene, lycopene, and lutein, which are found in colorful fruits and vegetables as well as flavonoids and polyphenols, which are abundant in tea, cocoa, and red wine.

Phytonutrients: Phytonutrients, also known as phytochemicals, are bioactive compounds found in plants that have antioxidant and anti-inflammatory properties. Examples include curcumin in turmeric, resveratrol in red grapes, and quercetin in onions and apples.

FOODS RICH IN ANTIOXIDANTS

Antioxidants play a crucial role in combating oxidative stress and inflammation in the body. Oxidative stress occurs when there is an imbalance between free radicals and antioxidants leading to damage to cells and tissues. By neutralizing free radicals, antioxidants help reduce inflammation and protect against chronic diseases.

Specific foods rich in antioxidants include:

- **Berries:** Berries such as blueberries, strawberries, raspberries, and blackberries are packed with antioxidants like anthocyanins, flavonoids, and vitamin C shown to reduce inflammation and oxidative stress, thus, potentially lower the risk of chronic diseases like heart disease and cancer.
- **Leafy greens:** Dark, leafy greens like spinach, kale, Swiss chard, and collard greens are rich in antioxidants such as vitamins A, C, and K, as well as phytonutrients like lutein and zeaxanthin. These antioxidants help protect cells from damage caused by free radicals and support overall health.
- **Nuts and seeds:** Almonds, walnuts, chia seeds, and flaxseeds are excellent sources of antioxidants like vitamin E, selenium, and polyphenols. These antioxidants have anti-inflammatory properties and may help reduce the risk of chronic diseases like diabetes and Alzheimer's disease.
- **Colorful fruits and vegetables:** Oranges, carrots, bell peppers, and tomatoes contain a variety of antioxidants like beta-carotene, lycopene, and vitamin C. These antioxidants help combat inflammation and support immune function.
- **Herbs and spices:** Turmeric, ginger, cinnamon, and garlic are just some of many herbs and spices rich in antioxidants with potent anti-inflammatory properties. These antioxidants help reduce inflammation and may alleviate symptoms of conditions like arthritis and IBD, as we explain in Chapter 11.

IMPACT OF CERTAIN FOODS ON INFLAMMATION

Diet plays a pivotal role in inflammation, as certain foods can either promote or mitigate inflammatory responses in the body.

Pro-inflammatory foods are those that can trigger or exacerbate inflammation in the body. These typically include highly processed foods, refined carbohydrates, sugary snacks and beverages, fried foods, and foods high in trans fats and saturated fats. Processed meats such as hot dogs and bacon are also considered inflammatory due to their high sodium and preservative content.

On the other hand, anti-inflammatory foods are those that help reduce inflammation in the body. These include fruits and vegetables rich in antioxidants, omega-3 fatty acids found in fatty fish like salmon and mackerel, nuts and seeds, whole grains, and healthy fats like olive oil and avocados. Herbs and spices like turmeric, ginger, and garlic are also known for their anti-inflammatory properties and can be incorporated into meals to help combat inflammation.

When you understand the impact of certain foods on inflammation, you can make informed dietary choices to support your overall health and well-being. Adopting a diet rich in anti-inflammatory foods while minimizing the intake of pro-inflammatory foods can help reduce chronic inflammation and lower the risk of associated health conditions.

PRO-INFLAMMATORY FOODS

Pro-inflammatory foods are those that can trigger or exacerbate inflammation in the body typically containing ingredients that promote the release of inflammatory mediators i.e., cytokines and prostaglandins. Here are some common pro-inflammatory foods and their potential effects:

- **Refined sugars and carbohydrates:** Desserts, candies, and sugary beverages can spike blood sugar levels leading to increased production of inflammatory cytokines. Additionally, refined carbohydrates like white bread, pasta, and pastries have a similar effect and may contribute to chronic inflammation, insulin resistance, and obesity.
- **Trans fats and saturated fats:** Trans fats—found in partially hydrogenated oils often used in processed and

fried foods—can promote inflammation by increasing levels of inflammatory markers like C-reactive protein and IL-6. Saturated fats commonly found in red meat, full-fat dairy products, and certain oils like palm oil may also contribute to inflammation and insulin resistance when consumed in excess.

- **Processed meats:** Processed meats such as bacon, sausage, deli meats, and hot dogs contain additives, preservatives, and high levels of sodium, which can trigger inflammation in the body. Moreover, these meats often undergo cooking methods like grilling or smoking, which can lead to the formation of pro-inflammatory compounds like advanced glycation end products.

- **Refined vegetable oils:** Vegetable oils like corn oil, soybean oil, and sunflower oil are high in omega-6 fatty acids, which —when consumed in excess and not balanced with omega-3 fatty acids—can promote inflammation. Their common use in processed foods, fried snacks, and baked goods contributes to the inflammatory load in the diet.

- **Artificial additives and preservatives:** Certain food additives and preservatives, such as monosodium glutamate, artificial sweeteners, and high-fructose corn syrup, have been linked to increased inflammation and oxidative stress in the body. These additives are commonly found in processed foods, fast food items, and convenience snacks.

Overall, consuming a diet high in pro-inflammatory foods can contribute to chronic low-grade inflammation, which is associated with an increased risk of various health conditions including cardiovascular disease, DM2, and certain cancers.

ANTI-INFLAMMATORY DIETS

In recent years, there has been a growing interest in anti-inflammatory diets as a means to manage inflammation and promote overall health. These diets focus on incorporating foods that have been shown to have anti-inflammatory properties while minimizing or avoiding pro-inflammatory foods.

There are several popular anti-inflammatory diets that individuals may choose to follow, each with its own specific guidelines and recommendations. These diets include the Mediterranean, DASH (Dietary Approaches to Stop Hypertension), Paleo, the Whole30 program, and the anti-inflammatory diet proposed by Dr. Andrew Weil, among others.

MEDITERRANEAN DIET

The Mediterranean diet is a dietary pattern inspired by the traditional eating habits of people living in countries bordering the Mediterranean Sea such as Greece, Italy, and Spain. It was first popularized in the 1960s by the American biologist Ancel Keys who observed the low rates of heart disease among populations in these regions and attributed it to their dietary habits (Lăcătușu et al., 2019).

The Mediterranean diet is characterized by an abundance of plant-based foods such as fruits, vegetables, whole grains, legumes, nuts, and seeds. The primary source of fat is olive oil—a key component of this diet. Additionally, moderate consumption of fish, poultry, dairy products (yogurt and cheese), and eggs is encouraged. Red meat is consumed sparingly, and sweets and processed foods are limited.

One of the distinctive features of the Mediterranean diet is its emphasis on consuming foods rich in monounsaturated and polyunsaturated fats, particularly omega-3 fatty acids found in fish and nuts. These fats have been shown to have anti-inflammatory properties and are believed to contribute to the diet's health benefits.

Research has consistently linked the Mediterranean diet to numerous health benefits including a reduced risk of heart disease, stroke, DM2, and certain cancers. Additionally, adherence to the Mediterranean diet has been associated with improved cognitive function, better weight management, and longevity (Widmer et al., 2015).

The Mediterranean diet is not just about the foods consumed but also encompasses lifestyle factors such as regular physical activity, shared meals with family and friends, and enjoyment of food in moderation. Its emphasis on whole, minimally processed foods and plant-based sources of nutrition aligns with principles of anti-inflammatory eating and has made it one of the most well-studied and recommended dietary patterns for promoting health and well-being.

THE DASH DIET

The DASH diet is a dietary pattern developed specifically to help lower blood pressure and prevent hypertension. It was initially designed by the National Heart, Lung, and Blood Institute (NHLBI) in collaboration with other research institutions (Campbell, 2017).

Emphasizing a balanced eating plan rich in fruits, vegetables, whole grains, lean proteins, and low-fat dairy products, it encourages reducing sodium intake and limiting foods high in saturated fats, cholesterol, and added sugars.

Key components of the DASH diet include:

- **Fruits and vegetables:** Aim to include a variety of colorful fruits and vegetables in your meals and snacks. These foods are high in vitamins, minerals, and antioxidants that support overall health.

- **Whole grains:** Choose whole grains such as brown rice, quinoa, oats, and whole wheat bread instead of refined grains, as they provide fiber, subsequently regulating blood sugar levels and promote heart health.
- **Lean proteins:** Opt for lean sources of protein such as poultry, fish, beans, lentils, and tofu. These foods are lower in saturated fat and provide essential nutrients like protein and iron.
- **Low-fat dairy:** Low-fat or fat-free milk, yogurt, and cheese to meet calcium needs while keeping saturated fat intake in check.
- **Limited sodium:** Reduce sodium intake by choosing fresh or minimally processed foods over packaged and processed foods. Season meals with herbs, spices, and citrus juices instead of salt.
- **Moderate alcohol consumption:** If you choose to drink alcohol, do so in moderation. Limit alcohol intake to one and two drinks per day for women and men, respectively.

The DASH diet has been shown to effectively lower blood pressure and reduce the risk of cardiovascular disease. It promotes overall heart health by emphasizing nutrient-rich foods and minimizing the intake of sodium and unhealthy fats. Following the DASH diet can also contribute to weight management, improved cholesterol levels, and better overall health outcomes.

THE PALEO DIET

The Paleo diet, also known as the Paleolithic or Caveman diet, is based on the premise of eating foods that were available to our ancient ancestors during the Paleolithic era. The diet emphasizes consuming whole, unprocessed foods that would have been hunted, fished, or gathered by early humans (Challa & Uppaluri, 2019).

Key principles of the Paleo diet include:

- **Focus on whole foods:** Lean meats, fish, seafood, fruits, vegetables, nuts, and seeds are encouraged. due to their wide range of nutrients and minimal processing.
- **Avoid processed foods:** Exclude processed foods including refined grains, sugars, and vegetable oils present in foods like bread, pasta, cereal, candy, and processed snacks.
- **Eliminate dairy and grains:** Dairy products like milk, cheese, yogurt, wheat, rice, oats and grains are not typically consumed on the Paleo diet. Instead, the focus is on alternative sources of calcium and carbohydrates such as leafy greens and starchy vegetables.
- **Limit legumes and beans:** Legumes and beans including lentils, chickpeas, and peanuts are restricted on the Paleo diet due to their potential anti-nutrient content i.e., they prevent absorption of vital nutrients. While some versions of the Paleo diet allow for limited legume consumption, others recommend avoiding them altogether.
- **Include healthy fats:** Healthy fats such as olive oil, coconut oil, avocado, and nuts are encouraged on the Paleo diet. These fats provide essential nutrients and can help promote satiety and overall health.
- **Emphasize protein:** Protein-rich foods like meat, poultry, fish, and eggs are staples of the Paleo diet, as they are essential muscle growth and repair.

The Paleo diet aims to mimic the dietary patterns of our ancient ancestors believed to have been free from many of the modern chronic diseases that plague society today. Advocates of the Paleo diet argue that it promotes weight loss, improves metabolic health, and reduces inflammation by eliminating processed foods and focusing on nutrient-dense whole foods. However, critics raise concerns about potential nutrient deficiencies, particularly in calcium and vitamin D, due to the exclusion of dairy products and grains. As with any diet, individual needs and preferences should be considered when deciding whether the Paleo diet is suitable.

WHOLE30 PROGRAM

The Whole30 program is a 30-day dietary reset designed to help individuals identify and eliminate potentially inflammatory or allergenic foods from their diet. Developed by Melissa Hartwig Urban and Dallas Hartwig in 2009, the program emphasizes whole, unprocessed foods and aims to promote better health, improve energy levels, and address various health concerns (Higuera, 2021).

Key principles of the Whole30 program include:

- **Elimination of certain foods:** During the 30-day period, participants are instructed to eliminate specific food groups —grains, dairy, legumes, added sugars, and alcohol— known to be potentially problematic for some individuals.
- **Focus on whole foods:** The program encourages the consumption of whole, nutrient-dense foods such as lean meats, fish, seafood, eggs, fruits, vegetables, nuts, and seeds. Processed foods, artificial additives, and preservatives are avoided.
- **No calorie counting or portion control:** Unlike some diet plans, the Whole30 program does not require participants to count calories or restrict portion sizes. Instead, the focus is on eating until satisfied and listening to hunger and fullness cues.
- **Strict 30-day** adherence: Participants are instructed to adhere strictly— to the program guidelines for the entire 30-day period without any deviations or "cheat" meals. This is intended to allow the body to fully reset and to

accurately assess the impact of different foods on individual health.

- **Gradual reintroduction of eliminated foods:** After completing the initial 30 days, participants gradually reintroduce eliminated foods one at a time over the course of several weeks. This process helps individuals identify any specific foods that may be causing adverse reactions or symptoms.

The Whole30 program is not intended as a long-term diet plan but rather as a short-term reset to help individuals identify and address potential food sensitivities, improve overall dietary habits, and promote healthier eating patterns. While some people may experience benefits such as improved energy, better digestion, and weight loss during the program, others may find it challenging to adhere to the strict guidelines or may not experience significant changes in their health outcomes.

As with any dietary intervention, it is essential to consult with a healthcare professional before starting the Whole30 program, especially if you have any underlying health conditions or concerns. Additionally, individuals should approach the program with realistic expectations and be mindful of their body's individual response to different foods.

DR. ANDRE WEIL ANTI-INFLAMMATORY DIET

The Dr. Andrew Weil anti-inflammatory Diet created by Dr. Andrew Weil—a renowned integrative medicine physician and wellness expert—is designed to reduce inflammation in the body and promote overall health and well-being. This diet is based on the premise that chronic inflammation contributes to the development of various diseases and health conditions including heart disease, diabetes, and autoimmune disorders (Weil, 2006).

Key principles of the Dr. Andrew Weil Anti-Inflammatory Diet include:

- **Emphasis on whole, nutrient-dense foods:** The diet encourages the consumption of whole foods that are rich in nutrients and antioxidants, such as fruits, vegetables, whole grains, legumes, nuts, and seeds. These foods provide essential vitamins, minerals, and phytonutrients that support overall health and reduce inflammation.
- **Focus on anti-inflammatory fats:** The diet emphasizes the importance of incorporating healthy fats into the diet, particularly those with anti-inflammatory properties. These include omega-3 fatty acids found in fatty fish like salmon, mackerel, and sardines, as well as in flaxseeds, chia seeds, and walnuts. Monounsaturated fats from sources like olive oil, avocado, and nuts are also encouraged.
- **Limitation of pro-inflammatory foods:** The diet advises reducing or eliminating foods that are known to promote inflammation in the body. These include processed foods, refined carbohydrates, sugary snacks and beverages, fried foods, and foods high in trans fats and saturated fats. Reducing the intake of these foods can help decrease inflammation and improve overall health.
- **Incorporation of anti-inflammatory herbs and spices:** The diet encourages the use of herbs and spices that have anti-inflammatory properties such as turmeric, ginger, garlic, cinnamon, and rosemary. These herbs and spices not only add flavor to meals but also provide additional health benefits by reducing inflammation and supporting immune function.
- **Moderation and balance:** While the Dr. Andrew Weil Anti-Inflammatory Diet promotes the consumption of nutrient-dense foods, it also emphasizes the importance of moderation and balance. It encourages mindful eating,

listening to hunger and fullness cues, and enjoying a variety of foods in appropriate portions.

MEAL PLANNING AND DIETARY TIPS

Designing meals that prioritize anti-inflammatory foods is an essential aspect of managing inflammation and promoting overall health. Here are some practical tips to help you create anti-inflammatory meals:

- **Focus on whole, minimally processed foods:** Choose whole grains like brown rice, quinoa, and oats, as well as lean proteins such as fish, poultry, tofu, and legumes. Incorporate plenty of fruits and vegetables aiming for a colorful variety to maximize nutrient intake.
- **Include omega-3 fatty acids:** Incorporate fatty fish like salmon, trout, and mackerel into your meals at least twice a week. Alternatively, add plant-based sources of omega-3s such as flaxseeds, chia seeds, and walnuts to salads, smoothies, or oatmeal.
- **Use healthy fats:** Opt for sources of healthy fats like olive oil, avocado oil, nuts, and seeds in cooking and meal preparation. These fats contain monounsaturated and polyunsaturated fatty acids, which have anti-inflammatory properties and support heart health.
- **Spice it up:** Use herbs and spices like turmeric, ginger, garlic, cinnamon, and rosemary to add flavor to your meals. Not only do these ingredients enhance the taste of your dishes, but they also contain anti-inflammatory compounds that can help reduce inflammation.
- **Limit added sugars and refined carbohydrates:** Minimize your intake of sugary beverages, processed snacks, and foods high in refined carbohydrates like white bread, pasta, and pastries. These foods can promote

inflammation and contribute to chronic health conditions.

- **Stay hydrated:** Drink plenty of water throughout the day to stay hydrated and support optimal bodily functions. Herbal teas and infused water can also provide hydration while offering additional antioxidants and anti-inflammatory benefits.
- **Plan ahead and prep meals:** Take time to plan your meals for the week considering your schedule and dietary preferences. Batch cooking and meal prepping can save time and ensure you have nutritious, anti-inflammatory meals readily available when you need them.

By incorporating these tips into your meal planning and preparation, you can create delicious and nourishing anti-inflammatory meals that support your overall health and well-being. Experiment with different ingredients and recipes to find combinations that work best for you and your dietary needs.

MINDFUL EATING PRACTICES

Given how busy our lives are, it is easy to rush through meals without paying much attention to what we're eating or how it makes us feel. However, practicing mindful eating can help us cultivate a greater awareness of our food choices, eating habits, and the sensations we experience while eating.

One key aspect of mindful eating is slowing down and savoring each bite. Instead of rushing through meals, take the time to appreciate the flavors, textures, and aromas of your food. Chew slowly and mindfully, allowing yourself to fully experience the taste sensations.

Another important component of mindful eating is listening to our body's hunger and fullness signals. Pay attention to when you are truly hungry and when you are satisfied. Learn to distinguish between physical hunger and emotional or situational hunger, and honor your body's cues accordingly.

Additionally, mindful eating involves being aware of the thoughts and emotions that arise during eating. Notice any judgments or criticisms you may have about your food choices, and practice self-compassion and acceptance instead. By cultivating a non-judgmental attitude towards food and eating, we can reduce stress and anxiety around mealtimes.

Practicing gratitude is another way to enhance mindful eating. Take a moment before eating to express gratitude for the food in front of you, as well as for the nourishment and sustenance it provides. This can help foster a sense of appreciation and connection with your food.

REFLECTIVE FOOD JOURNAL

To conclude our exploration of diet and inflammation, let us embark on a reflective food journaling activity. Take some time each day to jot down what you eat, how it makes you feel, and any observations about your eating habits. As you document your meals, pay attention to any patterns or correlations between certain foods and your overall well-being. Notice how your body responds to different foods —do some leave you feeling energized and vibrant, while others make you feel sluggish or bloated?

Additionally, consider incorporating mindfulness into your meals by practicing gratitude for the nourishment you receive and savoring each bite mindfully. Take note of the colors, textures, and flavors of your food, and pause to appreciate the journey it took from farm to table.

By keeping a food journal and practicing mindful eating, you will gain valuable insights into how your diet impacts inflammation and overall health. Use this information to make informed choices about the foods you consume, striving for a balanced, nutrient-rich diet that supports your well-being.

QUESTIONS TO PONDER ON

- How does my current diet make me feel physically and emotionally?
- Are there any patterns or correlations between certain foods and my energy levels or mood?
- What role does mindfulness play in my eating habits, and how can I incorporate more mindful eating practices into my daily life?
- Am I consuming a variety of nutrient-rich foods that support inflammation management and overall well-being?
- How can I make more informed choices about the foods I consume based on the insights gained from my food journaling activity?
- What steps can I take to create a more balanced and anti-inflammatory meal plan?
- How do I feel about the concept of superfoods, and how can I incorporate them into my diet?
- What changes can I make to my eating habits to support a healthier relationship with food and better manage inflammation in the long term?

Next up, in Chapter 11 we will explore the world of natural remedies and herbal supplements that have been used for centuries to promote health and well-being. Dive into the fascinating realm of botanical medicine and discover how these natural compounds can complement your lifestyle in managing inflammation and enhancing overall vitality.

CHAPTER II
NATURAL SUPPLEMENTS AND HERBS

*When I'm sore, ice is my best friend. It really works.
I take omega-3s every day, which helps with inflammation. And I try to eat things that won't inflame my
joints, like fresh fruits and veggies, lean protein, and
seafood.*

- Kerri Walsh

While many may overlook or distrust natural remedies, it is essential to recognize that numerous conventional medicines originate from natural sources. By exploring the science behind these botanical compounds, we can unlock their potential in managing inflammation and supporting overall health.

NATURAL SUPPLEMENTS AND INFLAMMATION

Using natural supplements as a complementary approach to manage chronic inflammation involves incorporating various botanical compounds and dietary supplements into one's daily routine. These supplements are derived from plants, herbs, and other natural sources—each offering unique anti-inflammatory properties. Unlike pharmaceutical drugs, natural supplements often work synergistically with the body's natural processes, promoting balance and supporting overall health without causing significant side effects.

One key advantage of natural supplements is their diverse range of bioactive compounds, including polyphenols, flavonoids, and phytochemicals, which exhibit potent anti-inflammatory effects. For example, curcumin, found in turmeric, is well-known for its anti-inflammatory and antioxidant properties. Similarly, omega-3 fatty acids—abundant in fish oil supplements—have been shown to reduce inflammation by inhibiting pro-inflammatory pathways in the body.

Moreover, natural supplements often contain vitamins, minerals, and other essential nutrients that play crucial roles in modulating the immune system and reducing inflammation. For instance, vitamin D—commonly obtained from sunlight exposure or supplements—has been linked to lower levels of inflammation in numerous studies.

It is important to note that while natural supplements can be beneficial for managing inflammation, they should not replace conventional medical treatments prescribed by healthcare professionals. Instead, they can complement existing therapies and lifestyle modifications to enhance their effectiveness. Additionally, it is essential to choose high-quality supplements from reputable sources to ensure safety and efficacy.

TURMERIC

Turmeric is a vibrant yellow spice commonly used in Indian cuisine and traditional medicine. It contains a bioactive compound called curcumin, which has been extensively studied for its potent anti-inflammatory properties. Curcumin works by targeting multiple pathways involved in inflammation, thereby helping to reduce inflammation in the body.

Research has shown that curcumin can inhibit the activity of inflammatory enzymes and molecules such as cyclooxygenase-2 (COX-2) and nuclear factor-kappa B (NF-kB), which play key roles in the inflammatory process. By blocking these pathways, curcumin helps to dampen the body's inflammatory response and alleviate symptoms associated with inflammation, such as pain and swelling (Peng et al., 2021).

In addition to its anti-inflammatory effects, curcumin is also a powerful antioxidant that can neutralize harmful free radicals that contribute to oxidative stress and damage to cells and tissues. This antioxidant activity further supports its role in combating inflammation and promoting overall health.

Turmeric can be incorporated into the diet in various ways such as adding it to curries, soups, stews, or smoothies. It can also be consumed in supplement form typically as a standardized extract containing higher concentrations of curcumin. However, it is important to note that the bioavailability of curcumin is relatively low, so consuming turmeric with black pepper containing piperine can enhance its absorption in the body.

OMEGA-3 FATTY ACIDS

Omega-3 fatty acids—abundant in fatty fish like salmon and available in fish oil supplements—are renowned for their potent anti-inflammatory properties. These essential fatty acids play a crucial role in modulating the body's inflammatory response by decreasing the production of pro-inflammatory molecules.

Studies have shown that omega-3 fatty acids, particularly eicosapentaenoic acid (EPA) and docosahexaenoic acid (DHA), can exert anti-inflammatory effects by competing with omega-6 fatty acids, which are known to promote inflammation. By incorporating omega-3 fatty acids into the diet, individuals may help rebalance the ratio of omega-6 to omega-3 fatty acids, thus, reducing inflammation and promoting overall health (Calder, 2013).

Furthermore, omega-3 fatty acids have been associated with various health benefits beyond their anti-inflammatory properties, including cardiovascular health, cognitive function, and mood regulation. Consuming fatty fish like salmon, mackerel, and sardines, or incorporating fish oil supplements, can be an effective way to increase omega-3 intake and support inflammatory balance.

GREEN TEA

Green tea is renowned for its abundant polyphenols, notably catechins, which boast antioxidant and anti-inflammatory properties. Consuming green tea regularly can potentially alleviate inflammation and bolster overall well-being.

Catechins—a type of polyphenols found in green tea—have been extensively studied for their health benefits and potent antioxidant properties like scavenging free radicals and reducing oxidative stress in the body. Additionally, catechins exhibit anti-inflammatory effects by modulating various inflammatory pathways and signaling molecules.

Research suggests that regular consumption of green tea may help mitigate inflammation associated with chronic diseases such as cardiovascular conditions, diabetes, and certain types of cancer. Furthermore, clinical studies have linked green tea to improvements in inflammatory markers of inflammation such as CRP levels (Zamani et al., 2023).

Incorporating green tea into your daily routine can be a simple yet effective way to support your body's natural defenses against inflammation. Whether enjoyed hot or cold, green tea offers a refreshing beverage option packed with potential health benefits. However, it is important to note that while green tea can complement a balanced diet and healthy lifestyle, it should not be viewed as a standalone solution for managing inflammation.

BOSWELLIA

Boswellia, commonly referred to as Indian frankincense, is a resin extracted from the Boswellia serrata tree. It contains bioactive compounds known as boswellic acids, which have demonstrated anti-inflammatory properties. These compounds work by targeting specific enzymes involved in the inflammatory cascade, such as 5-lipoxygenase (5-LOX).

Research suggests that boswellic acids can inhibit the activity of 5-LOX, an enzyme responsible for producing leukotrienes i.e., inflammatory mediators involved in various inflammatory conditions. By blocking this enzyme, boswellic acids help reduce the production of pro-inflammatory molecules, thereby attenuating the inflammatory response (Siddiqui, 2011).

Due to its anti-inflammatory effects, boswellia has been studied for its potential benefits in managing conditions associated with inflammation such as osteoarthritis and IBD. Studies have shown that boswellia supplementation may help alleviate symptoms such as joint pain and stiffness in individuals with osteoarthritis, as well as reduce inflammation in the gut mucosa of patients with IBD.

Boswellia supplements are available in various forms including capsules, extracts, and topical preparations. They are often used as complementary or alternative therapies for inflammatory conditions —either alone or in combination with other natural remedies. However, it is important to consult with a healthcare professional before using boswellia supplements, especially if you have underlying health issues or are taking medications, as they may interact with certain drugs or have potential side effects.

RESVERATROL

Resveratrol—a compound abundant in red grapes, berries, and peanuts—is celebrated for its potent antioxidant properties and anti-inflammatory effects. Research suggests that resveratrol may offer protection against chronic inflammatory diseases and age-related conditions.

Studies have highlighted the ability of resveratrol to combat inflammation by modulating various inflammatory pathways and reducing the production of pro-inflammatory molecules in the body. Additionally, resveratrol's antioxidant activity enables it to neutralize harmful free radicals, thereby mitigating oxidative stress and inflammation.

Consumption of resveratrol-rich foods may contribute to overall health and well-being by promoting a balanced inflammatory response. While further research is needed to fully understand the mechanisms and potential benefits, incorporating these nutritious foods into your diet can be a simple way to harness their anti-inflammatory properties.

However, it is important to note that while resveratrol shows promise as a natural anti-inflammatory agent, it should be consumed as part of a varied and balanced diet rather than relying solely on supplements.

ASHWAGANDHA

Ashwagandha—an adaptogenic herb deeply rooted in traditional Ayurvedic medicine—has garnered attention for its ability to help the body cope with stress and promote overall well-being i.e., to adapt. Beyond its stress-reducing properties, ashwagandha also boasts anti-inflammatory effects that may alleviate symptoms associated with inflammation.

Studies have highlighted the potential of ashwagandha to modulate the body's inflammatory response by inhibiting the activity of certain pro-inflammatory molecules and pathways. By exerting these anti-inflammatory actions, ashwagandha may offer relief from conditions characterized by chronic inflammation such as arthritis, asthma, and IBD (Mikulska et al., 2023).

Furthermore, ashwagandha's adaptogenic properties make it particularly beneficial for supporting the body's resilience to stress, which can often exacerbate inflammation. By helping to regulate the stress response, ashwagandha may indirectly contribute to the management of inflammation-related symptoms and promote overall health and well-being.

Ashwagandha supplements are available in various forms including capsules, powders, and tinctures, making it convenient for individuals to incorporate them into their daily routine. However, as with any herbal supplement, it is essential to choose high-quality products from reputable sources.

PRACTICAL IMPLEMENTATION

When integrating natural supplements into your daily routine, it is essential to establish a consistent schedule for consumption, as incorporating them into your morning or evening routine makes it easier to remember. You can set reminders on your phone or place the supplements in a visible location to prompt consumption. Additionally, pairing them with meals can enhance absorption and minimize any potential stomach discomfort.

It is important to recognize that responses to supplements can vary widely among individuals. Factors such as genetics, overall health status, and lifestyle habits can influence how your body reacts to different supplements. What works well for one person may not have the same effect for another. Therefore, it is essential to pay attention to your body's signals and work with healthcare professionals to find the right supplements for your unique needs.

It is crucial to consult with healthcare professionals before introducing new supplements into your routine, especially if you have existing health conditions or are taking medications. Your doctor or a registered dietitian can provide personalized guidance based on your medical history, current medications, and specific health goals. They can help you navigate potential interactions between supplements and medications, identify any contraindications, and ensure that your supplement regimen is safe and effective. By partnering with healthcare professionals, you can make informed decisions about incorporating supplements into your overall wellness plan.

As you begin taking natural supplements, it is crucial to monitor your body's response and adjust accordingly. Pay attention to any changes in symptoms, energy levels, or overall well-being. Keep track of your progress in a journal or on a digital platform to note any improvements or side effects. If you experience any adverse reactions or concerns, consult with a healthcare professional for personalized guidance.

QUESTIONS TO PONDER ON

- How do you currently manage inflammation in your daily life, and have you considered incorporating natural supplements and herbs into your routine?

- What specific symptoms of inflammation do you experience, and do you think natural remedies could offer relief?
- Have you ever tried any natural supplements or herbs for inflammation management, and if so, what were your experiences?
- What concerns or hesitations do you have about using natural supplements and herbs for inflammation, and how might you address them?
- Are you open to exploring the potential benefits of natural remedies alongside conventional treatments for inflammation, and why or why not?
- How do you plan to approach the integration of natural supplements and herbs into your wellness regimen, and what factors will you consider in your decision-making process?
- Have you discussed the possibility of using natural supplements and herbs with your healthcare provider, and what guidance have they offered?
- What lifestyle changes or modifications do you think could complement the use of natural supplements and herbs for inflammation management?
- Are there any specific natural remedies that you are particularly interested in exploring further, and why do they appeal to you?

In Chapter 12, we delve into groundbreaking advancements in medical treatment for inflammation exploring cutting-edge therapies, emerging technologies, and promising research that offer new hope and possibilities for managing chronic inflammatory conditions.

INNOVATIONS IN MEDICAL TREATMENT

The only way you multiply resources is with technology.
To really affect poverty, energy, health, education, or
anything else—there is no other way.

- Vinod Khosla

T his sentiment by Vinod Khosla underscores the pivotal role of innovation in addressing complex health challenges like inflammation. Just as technology has revolutionized various sectors from energy to education, it holds the promise of driving advancements in healthcare. By leveraging cutting-edge pharmaceuticals, biologics, and alternative therapies, we can harness the power of innovation to transform inflammation management and improve lives.

CURRENT MEDICAL TREATMENTS

Before we delve into the exciting realm of future innovations, let us take a moment to appreciate the medical treatments that are already making a difference in the realm of inflammation management. These existing therapies, ranging from pharmaceuticals to biologics, represent the culmination of years of research and development aimed at addressing inflammatory conditions. They serve as vital tools in the arsenal of healthcare providers, offering relief and hope to millions of individuals battling chronic inflammation. As we explore the landscape of current medical treatments, we recognize the significance of these established approaches in improving patient outcomes and paving the way for future advancements.

In the realm of conventional medicine, there are several established approaches to managing chronic inflammation—each tailored to address specific conditions and symptoms. Two commonly used classes of medications for inflammation management are non-steroidal anti-inflammatory drugs (NSAIDs) and corticosteroids. Others include:

NON-STEROIDAL ANTI-INFLAMMATORY DRUGS

NSAIDs are a class of medications commonly used to relieve pain and inflammation. They work by inhibiting enzymes called cyclooxygenases (COX), which play a key role in producing prostaglandins—substances that promote inflammation, pain, and fever. By blocking the action of these enzymes, NSAIDs help reduce inflammation and alleviate associated symptoms.

Examples of NSAIDs include ibuprofen, aspirin, and naproxen—among many. These medications are available over-the-counter or by prescription depending on their strength and formulation. While NSAIDs can be effective for short-term relief of inflammation and pain, long-term use may be associated with gastrointestinal issues, cardiovascular risks, and other side effects.

CORTICOSTEROIDS

Corticosteroids, also known simply as steroids, are synthetic drugs that mimic the effects of cortisol, a hormone naturally produced by the adrenal glands. Cortisol plays a crucial role in regulating inflammation and immune responses in the body. Corticosteroids work by suppressing inflammation and immune activity, thereby reducing swelling, pain, and other inflammatory symptoms.

These medications are available in various forms including oral tablets, injections, topical creams, and inhalers allowing for targeted delivery depending on the site and severity of inflammation. Common corticosteroids used to manage inflammation include prednisone, hydrocortisone, and dexamethasone. While corticosteroids can be highly effective in controlling inflammation, prolonged use may lead to adverse effects such as weight gain, osteoporosis, and increased susceptibility to infections.

In summary, NSAIDs and corticosteroids are integral components of conventional medical treatments for chronic inflammation. While they provide symptomatic relief and help manage inflammatory conditions, it is essential to use them judiciously under the guidance of a healthcare professional to minimize potential risks and optimize therapeutic benefits.

DISEASE-MODIFYING ANTI-RHEUMATIC DRUGS (DMARDS)

DMARDs are a class of medications used primarily to treat autoimmune diseases such as rheumatoid arthritis, psoriatic arthritis, and systemic lupus erythematosus. Unlike NSAIDs and corticosteroids, which provide symptomatic relief, DMARDs work to modify the underlying disease process, slowing or halting the progression of joint damage and inflammation. Examples of DMARDs include methotrexate, hydroxychloroquine, and sulfasalazine (Benjamin et al., 2022).

BIOLOGIC THERAPIES

Biologic therapies, also known as biologics, are a newer class of medications designed to target specific molecules involved in the inflammatory process. Biologics are commonly used in the treatment of autoimmune diseases and inflammatory conditions such as rheumatoid arthritis, psoriasis, and IBD. These medications are typically administered by injection or infusion and may include tumor necrosis factor (TNF) inhibitors, interleukin inhibitors, and other targeted therapies.

IMMUNOMODULATORS

Immunomodulators are medications that help regulate the immune system and reduce inflammation by targeting immune cells and pathways involved in the inflammatory response. These medications are used in various autoimmune and inflammatory conditions including Crohn's disease, ulcerative colitis, and multiple sclerosis. Examples of immunomodulators include azathioprine, cyclosporine, and tacrolimus.

TOPICAL TREATMENTS

Topical treatments such as corticosteroid creams, gels, and ointments are commonly used to manage localized inflammation associated with skin conditions such as eczema, psoriasis, and dermatitis. These medications are applied directly to the affected skin area, thus, providing targeted relief from itching, redness, and swelling.

IMMUNOTHERAPY

Immunotherapy involves the use of medications that modulate the immune system to reduce inflammation and improve disease outcomes. This approach may include allergen immunotherapy for allergic conditions, cytokine inhibitors for certain inflammatory diseases, and other specialized treatments aimed at restoring immune balance.

CYTOKINE INHIBITORS

Cytokine inhibitors are a class of medications that target specific cytokines—signaling proteins involved in the inflammatory response. By blocking the action of these cytokines, cytokine inhibitors help reduce inflammation and alleviate the symptoms of various inflammatory conditions. Examples of cytokine inhibitors include TNF inhibitors, interleukin inhibitors, and Janus kinase (JAK) inhibitors. JAK inhibitors are a type of medication that blocks the activity of Janus kinases, enzymes involved in the signaling pathways of various cytokines and growth factors. By inhibiting JAK enzymes, these medications help reduce inflammation and modulate the immune response. JAK inhibitors are used in the treatment of inflammatory conditions such as RA, psoriatic arthritis, and IBD (Zhang & An, 2007).

LIMITATIONS AND CHALLENGES

While current medical treatments play a crucial role in managing chronic inflammation, they are not without limitations and potential side effects. NSAIDs and corticosteroids, for example, can cause gastrointestinal problems, an increased risk of cardiovascular events, and other adverse effects with long-term use. Similarly, biologic medications such as cytokine inhibitors and JAK inhibitors may be associated with risks such as increased susceptibility to infections, liver toxicity, and immune-related complications.

Furthermore, some patients may not respond adequately to conventional treatments, or they may experience only partial relief from their symptoms. Additionally, the high cost of certain biologic medications may limit access for some patients, leading to disparities in healthcare.

The need for ongoing research and innovation in inflammation management is evident. There is a growing understanding of the complex mechanisms underlying chronic inflammation, and new therapeutic targets are continually being identified. Advances in biotechnology, pharmacology, and immunology are paving the way for the development of novel treatments with improved efficacy, safety, and tolerability profiles.

Moreover, personalized medicine approaches such as biomarker-based therapy selection and genetic testing hold promise for optimizing treatment outcomes and minimizing adverse effects. Collaborative efforts between clinicians, researchers, pharmaceutical companies, and regulatory agencies are essential to drive innovation and address the unmet needs of patients with inflammatory diseases. By harnessing the power of technology, research, and collaboration, we can strive towards more effective, personalized, and accessible treatments for chronic inflammation.

EMERGING THERAPIES

As our understanding of the underlying mechanisms of chronic inflammation deepens, there is a growing interest in developing more targeted and personalized treatment options. Emerging therapies aim to address the specific pathways and molecules involved in the inflammatory process, therefore, offering the potential for improved efficacy and reduced side effects compared to traditional treatments.

NF-KB INHIBITORS

Nuclear factor kappa-light-chain-enhancer of activated B cells (NF-kB) is a transcription factor that plays a key role in regulating genes involved in inflammation, immunity, and cell survival. NF-kB inhibitors are medications that target the NF-kB signaling pathway, thereby reducing the production of pro-inflammatory molecules and dampening the inflammatory response. These inhibitors may be used in the treatment of various inflammatory diseases including RA, IBD, and psoriasis. However, the development of specific NF-kB inhibitors for clinical use is still ongoing, and more research is needed to fully understand their efficacy and safety profile.

CLUSTERED REGULARLY INTERSPACED SHORT PALINDROMIC REPEATS AND CRISPR-ASSOCIATED PROTEIN 9

Advances in gene editing technologies, particularly CRISPR-Cas9, have revolutionized the field of medicine by offering unprecedented precision and control over genetic modifications. CRISPR-Cas9 allows researchers to precisely target and edit specific genes within the genome, including those associated with inflammation (Tavakoli et al., 2021).

In the context of chronic inflammation, researchers are exploring the potential of CRISPR-Cas9 to directly target genes that regulate inflammatory pathways. By selectively modifying these genes, it becomes possible to modulate the immune response and dampen excessive inflammation in a highly targeted manner.

One of the key advantages of CRISPR-Cas9 is its ability to tailor interventions to individual genetic profiles. By analyzing an individual's genetic makeup, clinicians can identify specific genetic variations that contribute to inflammation susceptibility or severity. With this information, CRISPR-Cas9 can be used to target and modify the relevant genes, thus, offering personalized interventions tailored to the unique genetic characteristics of each patient.

Moreover, CRISPR-Cas9 holds promise for addressing underlying genetic defects or mutations that predispose individuals to chronic inflammatory conditions. By correcting these genetic abnormalities, CRISPR-based therapies have the potential to not only alleviate symptoms but also address the root cause of inflammation leading to more sustainable and long-lasting therapeutic outcomes (Liu et al., 2021).

Overall, the shift toward more targeted and personalized treatment options represents a paradigm shift in the management of chronic inflammation. By tailoring therapies to the specific molecular pathways and genetic factors driving inflammation in each patient, clinicians can optimize treatment outcomes while minimizing the risk of adverse effects. However, further research and clinical trials are needed to validate the efficacy and safety of these emerging therapies and to bring them to the forefront of clinical practice.

ALTERNATIVE THERAPIES AND INTEGRATIVE APPROACHES

Non-traditional and complementary therapies offer alternative approaches to inflammation management often focusing on holistic healing and addressing underlying imbalances in the body. Acupuncture and homeopathy are two such therapies that have gained popularity for their potential benefits in reducing inflammation and promoting overall well-being.

Acupuncture is a traditional Chinese medicine practice that involves the insertion of thin needles into specific points on the body to stimulate energy flow and restore balance. It is believed to work by regulating the body's energy, or Qi, and promoting the release of natural pain-relieving chemicals. In terms of inflammation management, acupuncture may help by reducing pain and inflammation, as well as by modulating the immune response (Zhu, 2014).

Homeopathy is a holistic system of medicine based on the principle of "like cures like," where highly diluted substances that cause symptoms in healthy individuals are used to stimulate the body's natural healing processes. Homeopathic remedies are prepared through a process of dilution and succussion (energetically shaking), which is believed to enhance their healing properties. While the mechanism of action of homeopathy is not fully understood, proponents suggest that it works by stimulating the body's vital force and restoring balance on a physical, mental, and emotional level.

Both acupuncture and homeopathy offer individualized treatment approaches tailored to each person's unique needs and constitution. They may be used alone or in conjunction with conventional medical treatments to support inflammation management and promote overall health and well-being. However, it is essential to consult with qualified practitioners and healthcare professionals to ensure the safe and appropriate use of these therapies, especially if you have underlying health conditions or are taking medications.

PATIENT-CENTRIC APPROACHES

Patient-centric approaches prioritize the individual needs, preferences, and values of patients in the design and delivery of healthcare services. In the context of innovative treatments for inflammation, patient-centric care emphasizes the importance of involving patients as active participants in their treatment journey. This approach recognizes that patients have unique experiences, goals, and priorities, which should guide treatment decisions and interventions.

Shared decision-making is a key aspect of patient-centric care, where healthcare providers and patients collaborate to make informed decisions about treatment options based on the best available evidence and the patient's preferences and values. This collaborative process allows patients to contribute their insights, concerns, and preferences to the decision-making process, consequently empowering them to play an active role in their own care.

Patient involvement in treatment plans goes beyond simply following medical recommendations; it involves engaging patients in discussions about their treatment goals, potential benefits and risks, and alternative approaches. By fostering open communication and mutual respect between patients and healthcare providers, patient-centric care ensures that treatment decisions align with patients' values and preferences leading to more personalized and meaningful care experiences.

Innovative treatments for inflammation often require a multidisciplinary approach involving various healthcare professionals, researchers, and patients working together to explore new therapies, technologies, and interventions. Patient engagement in research and clinical trials is also essential for ensuring that treatments are not only effective but also acceptable, feasible, and accessible to those who need them.

QUESTIONS TO PONDER ON

- What are the potential benefits and limitations of non-traditional and complementary therapies, such as acupuncture and homeopathy, in the context of chronic inflammation?
- How can patient-centric approaches improve the overall effectiveness and patient experience of innovative treatments for inflammation?
- What role should patients play in shared decision-making processes when considering various treatment options for chronic inflammation?
- In what ways might advancements in medical treatments impact the future landscape of inflammation management,

and how can individuals stay informed about these developments?

Chapter 13 offers a comprehensive guide to creating a personalized approach to inflammation management. From integrating lifestyle modifications and dietary changes to exploring innovative medical treatments, this final chapter empowers you to craft your own effective strategies for combating chronic inflammation and enhancing overall well-being.

CHAPTER 13
BUILDING YOUR ANTI-INFLAMMATORY PLAN

*Self-compassion and a sense of being your biggest cheer-
leader should always be the underlying causes of
anything you do for your health and wellness. Why? You
can't heal a body you hate.*

- Will Cole

Crafting your anti-inflammatory plan is a journey as unique as you are. There is no one-size-fits-all approach because our experiences, needs, and goals vary. In this chapter, we will guide you through a step-by-step process to create a personalized anti-inflammatory plan tailored to your lifestyle, preferences, and health objectives.

STEP-BY-STEP GUIDE

ASSESSING CURRENT LIFESTYLE AND HABITS

- Begin by examining your daily routines including your dietary choices, exercise habits, work schedule, and leisure activities.
- Take note of any habits that may contribute to inflammation such as consuming processed foods high in sugar or trans fats, leading a sedentary lifestyle, or experiencing chronic stress.
- Reflect on how these habits impact your overall well-being and whether they align with your health goals.

IDENTIFYING POTENTIAL INFLAMMATORY TRIGGERS

- Pay attention to how certain foods, activities, or environmental factors affect your body and mood. Notice any patterns or correlations between your habits and symptoms of inflammation.
- Consider factors such as food sensitivities or allergies, exposure to toxins or pollutants, lack of sleep, or unresolved emotional stress.
- Keep a journal to track your symptoms and record any triggers you identify. This can help you pinpoint specific areas for improvement and develop strategies to address them.

EVALUATING PERSONAL HEALTH GOALS

Take time to reflect on and clarify your personal health goals and priorities. Consider what aspects of your well-being are most important to you, whether it is improving energy levels, managing chronic conditions, or achieving greater mental clarity. One way to set yourself up for success is adapting your goals to be specific, measurable, achievable, relevant, and time-bound i.e. SMART:

Specific: Define clear and specific anti-inflammatory goals that outline exactly what you want to achieve. For example, rather than setting a vague goal like "eat healthier," specify that you aim to incorporate more fruits and vegetables into your daily meals or reduce your intake of processed foods.

Measurable: Establish measurable criteria for tracking your progress toward your anti-inflammatory goals. This could involve quantifying your dietary changes by aiming to consume a certain number of servings of vegetables per day or reducing your intake of added sugars to a specific amount.

Achievable: Set goals that are realistic and attainable based on your current lifestyle, resources, and circumstances. Consider your individual strengths and limitations when determining what you can feasibly accomplish. Break larger goals into smaller, manageable steps to increase your likelihood of success.

Relevant: Ensure that your anti-inflammatory goals align with your overarching health priorities and values. Focus on areas of your life where reducing inflammation can have the greatest impact on your well-being and QOL. Tailor your goals to address your specific inflammatory triggers and health concerns.

Time-bound: Establish a timeframe for achieving your anti-inflammatory goals to create a sense of urgency and accountability. Set deadlines or milestones to work toward within designated time periods, whether it is weeks, months, or longer-term goals. Regularly reassess and adjust your timeline as needed to stay on track and maintain momentum.

By applying the SMART criteria to your anti-inflammatory goals, you can create a roadmap for success that is tailored to your individual needs and preferences. This strategic approach helps you stay focused, motivated, and empowered to make meaningful changes in your lifestyle and health habits.

PRIORITIZING GOALS

- **Impact on well-being:** Evaluate the potential impact of each goal on your overall health and well-being. Identify goals that address key areas of inflammation management and have the greatest potential to improve your QOL. Consider factors such as reducing pain and discomfort, enhancing energy levels, improving mood, and supporting long-term health outcomes.
- **Inflammatory triggers:** Prioritize goals that directly target your identified inflammatory triggers and risk factors. Focus on addressing lifestyle habits, dietary choices, environmental factors, and other contributors to inflammation that have the most significant influence on your health. By targeting these triggers, you can effectively reduce inflammation and mitigate its negative effects on your body.
- **Feasibility and sustainability:** Assess the feasibility and sustainability of each goal in the context of your current lifestyle, resources, and commitments. Choose goals that are realistic and attainable within your available time, energy, and financial constraints. Avoid setting overly ambitious goals that may lead to burnout or discouragement. Instead, opt for gradual, sustainable changes that can be maintained over the long term.

- **Phased approach:** Consider adopting a phased approach to goal prioritization to prevent overwhelm and facilitate steady progress. Divide your goals into smaller, manageable milestones or phases that can be tackled sequentially. Start with high-priority goals that address immediate health concerns or critical areas of inflammation, then gradually incorporate additional goals as you build momentum and confidence.

TRACKING PROGRESS

- **Start a journal:** Begin by setting up a journal where you can record important details about your daily habits including your dietary choices, physical activity, stress levels, and any symptoms or changes in your health. Consider using a notebook, digital app, or even a simple spreadsheet to organize your entries.
- **Document your choices:** Make it a habit to document what you eat and drink throughout the day, while also noting the types of foods you consume, portion sizes, and any noticeable reactions or symptoms you experience after eating. Record details about your physical activity such as the duration and intensity of your workouts, as well as any relaxation techniques or stress management strategies you incorporate into your routine.
- **Use templates:** To make tracking easier, consider using templates or examples provided in resources or apps designed for health journaling. These tools may offer structured formats for recording meals, exercise sessions, mood changes, and other relevant information, hence, simplifying the identification of patterns and trends over time.
- **Be consistent:** Aim to make journaling a consistent part of your daily routine. Set aside a few minutes each day to

update your journal, reflecting on your experiences and observations. Consistency is key to gaining valuable insights into how your habits and choices impact your inflammation levels and overall health.

- **Weight and waist circumference:** Regularly monitoring your weight and waist circumference can provide valuable insights into changes in your body composition and overall health. Keep track of these measurements over time to assess whether your lifestyle modifications are leading to positive outcomes.
- **Inflammatory markers:** Consider discussing with your healthcare provider the possibility of testing for inflammatory markers, such as CRP or ESR. These markers can help gauge the level of inflammation in your body and provide additional data points for evaluating the effectiveness of your anti-inflammatory strategies.
- **Regular health assessments:** Make it a priority to schedule regular health assessments with your healthcare provider to monitor your progress and address any concerns or questions you may have. These assessments may include blood tests, physical examinations, and discussions about your overall well-being.

STAYING MOTIVATED

To maintain motivation on your anti-inflammatory journey, it is important to celebrate milestones along the way, no matter how small they may seem.

Celebrating milestones allows you to acknowledge the progress you have made towards your goals. Whether it is sticking to your dietary plan for a week or achieving a new personal best in your exercise routine, taking the time to recognize your accomplishments boosts your confidence and motivation.

Celebrating milestones provides positive reinforcement for your efforts, making you more likely to continue working towards your goals. It reminds you that your hard work is paying off and encourages you to stay committed to your anti-inflammatory plan.

Each milestone you celebrate becomes a stepping stone to the next, creating momentum towards your ultimate objectives. By breaking your journey into smaller, achievable goals and celebrating each one, you build confidence and motivation to tackle the next challenge.

Now, here are some ideas for how you can reward yourself and celebrate your achievements:

- Treat yourself to a relaxing spa day or massage to unwind and recharge.
- Enjoy a healthy, indulgent meal at your favorite restaurant as a reward for sticking to your dietary plan.
- Splurge on a new workout outfit or piece of fitness equipment to motivate yourself to stay active.
- Plan a fun outing or activity with friends or loved ones to celebrate reaching a milestone together.
- Take time to reflect on your progress and write yourself a congratulatory note or journal entry to acknowledge your hard work and determination.

CULTIVATING INTRINSIC MOTIVATION

Intrinsic motivation refers to the internal desire or drive to engage in an activity for its own sake rather than for external rewards or pressures. It arises from personal enjoyment, interest, or satisfaction derived from the activity itself. In the context of embarking on an anti-inflammatory journey, intrinsic motivation is essential because:

- **Sustainability:** External motivators, such as rewards or punishments, may provide temporary compliance but often fail to sustain long-term behavior change. Intrinsic motivation, on the other hand, fuels sustained commitment and enthusiasm for making healthier choices, even in the absence of external incentives.

- **Autonomy:** Intrinsic motivation empowers you to take ownership of your health and well-being, therefore, make choices aligned with your values, preferences, and goals. This sense of autonomy fosters a deeper sense of personal responsibility and investment in the journey toward inflammation management.
- **Resilience:** When faced with challenges or setbacks, intrinsic motivation serves as a resilient force, driving you to persist in their efforts and overcome obstacles. The inherent satisfaction derived from pursuing meaningful goals helps you bounce back from setbacks and stay on course despite adversity.
- **Inherent Fulfillment:** Engaging in activities driven by intrinsic motivation brings inherent satisfaction and fulfillment, enhancing overall well-being beyond the specific goals of inflammation management. By deriving pleasure and fulfillment from the journey itself, you are more likely to maintain motivation and enjoyment throughout the process.

Here is how you can cultivate intrinsic motivation:

Connect with Personal Values: Reflect on your core values and how your health and well-being align with them. By recognizing the intrinsic importance of taking care of yourself, you can tap into a deeper sense of motivation rooted in personal fulfillment and alignment with your values.

Find Joy in the Journey: Shift your focus from solely achieving end goals to finding joy in the process of making positive changes. Embrace the small victories along the way, celebrate your progress, and cultivate gratitude for the opportunity to prioritize your health and well-being.

Mindset Shift: Adopt a growth mindset, recognizing that setbacks and challenges are natural parts of any journey toward improvement. View obstacles as opportunities for learning and growth rather than barriers to success. By reframing your perspective, you can maintain resilience and stay committed to your anti-inflammatory goals.

OVERCOMING CHALLENGES

Having a plan on paper may seem straightforward and easy, akin to taking a leisurely stroll through the park. However, the reality is often quite different. Like any other journey, embarking on an anti-inflammatory plan comes with its own set of challenges and hurdles to overcome. It is important to acknowledge and prepare for these obstacles in order to navigate them effectively. Here are some common challenges you may encounter:

- **Time constraints:** Balancing work, family responsibilities, social commitments, and self-care can be challenging. Finding time to prepare nutritious meals, exercise regularly, and practice stress-reducing activities may seem daunting amidst a busy schedule.
- **Social pressures:** Social gatherings, parties, and dining out can present temptations and peer pressure to deviate from healthy eating habits. It can be challenging to stick to an anti-inflammatory diet while navigating social situations where unhealthy foods are prevalent.
- **Unexpected setbacks:** Life is unpredictable, and unexpected events such as illness, injury, or personal crises can disrupt even the best-laid plans. Coping with setbacks

while staying committed to the anti-inflammatory journey requires resilience and adaptability.

- **Emotional eating:** Stress, boredom, or other emotional triggers can lead to cravings for comfort foods that are high in sugar, fat, and processed ingredients. Overcoming emotional eating habits and making mindful choices in moments of vulnerability can be a significant challenge.
- **Lack of support:** Without a supportive environment or network, maintaining motivation and adherence to an anti-inflammatory plan can be difficult. Lack of encouragement or understanding from friends, family, or healthcare providers may hinder progress.

Here are some strategies to overcome common challenges in adhering to an anti-inflammatory plan:

TIME CONSTRAINTS

- **Prioritize:** Identify your top health goals and prioritize activities that support them.
- **Schedule:** Block out dedicated time slots for meal planning, exercise, and self-care in your calendar.
- **Batch cooking:** Prepare large batches of healthy meals in advance and freeze individual portions for quick and convenient meals during busy days.
- **Multitask:** Find opportunities to combine activities such as listening to health podcasts while exercising or meal prepping with family members.

SOCIAL PRESSURES

- **Communicate:** Explain your dietary preferences and health goals to friends and family to gain their understanding and support.

- **Offer alternatives:** Bring your own nutritious dishes to social gatherings or suggest restaurants with healthier options.
- **Stay assertive:** Politely decline unhealthy food offerings and focus on enjoying the company rather than the food.

UNEXPECTED SETBACKS

- **Flexibility:** Be adaptable and willing to adjust your plan when unexpected challenges arise.
- **Self-compassion:** Practice self-compassion and forgiveness if you veer off track temporarily. Remember that setbacks are normal and part of the learning process.
- **Seek support:** Reach out to friends, family, or support groups for encouragement and guidance during difficult times.

EMOTIONAL EATING

- **Mindful awareness:** Tune into your emotions and recognize triggers for emotional eating. Practice mindfulness techniques to pause and reflect before acting on cravings.
- **Healthy coping strategies:** Develop alternative coping mechanisms for managing stress or emotional distress, such as meditation, journaling, or engaging in hobbies.
- **Stock healthy options:** Keep nutritious snacks readily available to satisfy hunger and prevent impulsive eating of unhealthy foods.

LACK OF SUPPORT

Educate: Share information about the benefits of an anti-inflammatory lifestyle with your support network to garner understanding and encouragement.

Find like-minded individuals: Seek out online communities, support groups, or local meetups where you can connect with others who share similar health goals.

Work with a healthcare provider: Seek guidance from a healthcare provider or nutritionist who can offer personalized advice and support tailored to your needs.

BUILDING RESILIENCE

Building resilience is essential for overcoming challenges and staying committed to your anti-inflammatory plan. Here are some strategies to help you cultivate resilience and navigate setbacks effectively:

- **Adopt a growth mindset:** Embrace challenges as opportunities for growth rather than viewing them as insurmountable obstacles. Focus on learning from setbacks and using them to fuel personal development and progress.
- **Practice self-compassion:** Be kind to yourself during difficult times and recognize that setbacks are a natural part of the journey toward better health. Treat yourself with the same empathy and understanding that you would offer to a friend facing similar challenges.
- **Set realistic expectations:** Avoid setting overly ambitious goals that may set you up for disappointment. Instead, break down your goals into smaller, achievable steps, and celebrate each milestone along the way.

- **Stay flexible:** Recognize that plans may need to be adjusted in response to unexpected challenges or changes in circumstances. Be willing to adapt and modify your approach as needed while staying focused on your long-term goals.
- **Focus on progress, not perfection:** Shift your mindset from striving for perfection to embracing progress. Celebrate small victories and improvements along the way, even if they may seem insignificant compared to your ultimate goals.

SAMPLE DAY IN YOUR ANTI-INFLAMMATORY PLAN

The following sample day is just a template and should serve as inspiration for designing your personalized anti-inflammatory plan.

MORNING

Start your day with a nourishing turmeric-infused smoothie, harnessing its anti-inflammatory properties to kick-start your morning routine.

Take 10 min to practice mindfulness or deep breathing exercises, hence, setting a positive and focused tone for the day ahead.

AFTERNOON

Opt for a balanced lunch featuring omega-3-rich salmon accompanied by leafy greens and a variety of colorful vegetables to support your body's anti-inflammatory response.

Take advantage of a break by going for a short walk, thus, promoting physical activity and reducing stress levels to maintain overall well-being.

EVENING

Incorporate anti-inflammatory herbs such as ginger and garlic into your dinner, therefore, enhancing both flavor and health benefits.

Wind down your evening with a relaxing activity, whether it's reading a book, practicing gentle stretching, or engaging in another calming pursuit to prepare for a restful night's sleep.

THROUGHOUT THE DAY

Stay hydrated by drinking plenty of water and incorporating herbal teas known for their anti-inflammatory properties.

Snack on nuts and berries between meals to gain the sustained energy and antioxidant benefits they offer.

Tailor your plan according to your individual preferences, dietary needs, and lifestyle constraints while aligning it with your unique journey toward inflammation management and overall well-being.

VOICES AGAINST THE SILENT FIRE

"Never doubt that a small group of thoughtful, committed citizens can change the world. Indeed, it is the only thing that ever has."

— MARGARET MEAD

As you close the last chapter of *Inflammation The Silent Fire: Combat Chronic Inflammation With a Science-Backed Approach,* reflect on the knowledge and personal experiences you've gained. This book isn't just a compendium of scientific facts—it's a call to share your unique journey and insights into dealing with chronic inflammation.

Your story is powerful, potentially a guiding light for others in the shadows. Would you consider sharing your insights and reflections to help a stranger you may never meet?

When you write a review, you help:

- Guide others by illustrating practical strategies that have worked.
- Support the community by showing that no one is alone in this struggle.
- Inspire resilience through your personal successes and challenges.

Leaving a review is a simple yet impactful way to contribute, and it also nets you great Karma points!

Please take a moment to leave your review on Amazon at this link:

https://www.amazon.com/review/review-your-purchases/?asin=BOD2B5HCTB

Each review helps more than you might think. It not only assists in better positioning the book on Amazon through its complex algorithms but also makes it more likely to be seen and purchased by those who desperately need this information.

Thank you for considering sharing your experience. Together, our stories and voices can provide comfort, inspiration, and invaluable guidance to those still navigating the complexities of chronic inflammation.

With sincere appreciation,

Dr. Carly Stewart - DPT

P.S. - Remember, your story does more than review a book; it educates, it empathizes, and it empowers. Share your unique perspective, and let's help others discover the tools they need to manage their health effectively. Your words light up dark corners and offer hope to those on similar paths.

CONCLUSION:
EMBRACING YOUR
ANTI-INFLAMMATORY
JOURNEY

Health is like money, we never have a true idea of its value until we lose it.

- Josh Billings

As we close this book, let us take a moment to reflect on the valuable insights we have gained and the transformative journey we have embarked upon together. Throughout these pages, we have explored the intricate relationship between lifestyle choices, inflammation, and overall well-being. Here are some key takeaways to remember:

- **Lifestyle modifications matter:** Your daily habits—from diet and exercise to stress management and sleep—play a pivotal role in influencing inflammatory responses in your body.
- **A holistic approach is key:** Embracing a holistic approach that encompasses all aspects of health—physical, mental,

and emotional—is essential for managing chronic inflammation effectively.

- **Personalized care is vital:** There is no one-size-fits-all solution. Your anti-inflammatory plan should be tailored to your unique needs, preferences, and circumstances.
- **Small changes yield big results:** Even simple adjustments to your lifestyle can make a significant difference over time. Consistency is key—small, sustainable changes add up to meaningful improvements in inflammation management.
- **Empowerment through knowledge:** By understanding the impact of various lifestyle factors on inflammation, you empower yourself to make informed choices that support your health and well-being.

Now, it is time to put your newfound knowledge into practice. Take the lessons learned from this book and apply them to your daily life. Start by setting achievable goals, whether it is incorporating more anti-inflammatory foods into your diet, establishing a regular exercise routine, or prioritizing stress-relieving activities.

Remember, progress may not always be linear, and setbacks are a natural part of the journey. Approach each day with patience, kindness, and perseverance. Celebrate your successes, no matter how small, and learn from any challenges you encounter along the way.

We invite you to share your experiences and insights with us. Leave a review of the book and join the conversation by sharing your journey with others. Together, we can support and inspire each other to lead healthier, more vibrant lives.

As you close this book and step into the world beyond these pages, remember this: You hold the power to shape your health, happiness, and future. Embrace the journey of self-discovery, harness the tools you have gained, and forge ahead with confidence and determination. With each mindful choice, each step toward well-being, you are creating a life rich in vitality and resilience. Trust in your ability to thrive, and let your journey toward optimal health be a testament to the strength of your spirit. You are capable, resilient, and deserving of a life filled with vibrancy and joy. So go forth, dear friend, and live fully, live vibrantly, and live well.

REFERENCES

Belluz, J. (2016, January 9). Most "anti-inflammation" diets are overkill. Tom brady's is a case in point. *Vox.* https://www.vox.com/2016/1/9/10738744/tom-brady-inflammation-diet

Benjamin, O., Bansal, P., Goyal, A., & Lappin, S. L. (2022, July 4). Disease modifying anti-rheumatic drugs (DMARD). *StatPearls Publishing.* https://www.ncbi.nlm.nih.gov/books/NBK507863/

Beurel, E., Toups, M., & Nemeroff, C. B. (2020). The Bidirectional relationship of depression and inflammation: Double trouble. *Neuron, 107*(2). https://doi.org/10.1016/j.neuron.2020.06.002

Calder, P. C. (2013). Omega-3 polyunsaturated fatty acids and inflammatory processes: nutrition or pharmacology? *British Journal of Clinical Pharmacology, 75*(3), 645–662. https://doi.org/10.1111/j.1365-2125.2012.04374.x

Campbell, A. P. (2017). DASH eating plan: An eating pattern for diabetes management. *Diabetes Spectrum, 30*(2), 76–81. https://doi.org/10.2337/ds16-0084

Cerqueira, É., Marinho, D. A., Neiva, H. P., & Lourenço, O. (2020). Inflammatory effects of high and moderate intensity exercise—a systematic review. *Frontiers in Physiology, 10.* https://doi.org/10.3389/fphys.2019.01550

Challa, H. J., & Uppaluri, K. R. (2019, May 29). Paleolithic Diet. *StatPearls Publishing.* https://www.ncbi.nlm.nih.gov/books/NBK482457/

Chen, L., Deng, H., Cui, H., Fang, J., Zuo, Z., Deng, J., Li, Y., Wang, X., & Zhao, L. (2017). Inflammatory responses and inflammation-associated diseases in organs. *Oncotarget, 9*(6), 7204–7218. https://doi.org/10.18632/oncotarget.23208

Cole, W. (2019, October 15).*The inflammation spectrum: Find your food triggers and reset your system.* Avery.

DC, D. E. G. (2011, July 14). *The 50 best quotes about health & nutrition.* Dr. Group's Healthy Living Articles. https://explore.globalhealing.com/quotes-about-health/

Edward Bullmore quotes. (n.d.). *The inflamed mind quotes by Edward Bullmore.* Goodreads. https://www.goodreads.com/work/quotes/61739028-the-inflamed-mind

Famous Quotes & Sayings. (n.d.). *Top 23 lymph quotes: Famous quotes & sayings about lymph.* Quotestats. https://quotestats.com/topic/lymph-quotes/

Famous Quotes & Sayings. (n.d.). *Top 41 quotes about inflammation: Famous quotes & sayings about inflammation.* Quotestats. https://quotestats.com/topic/quotes-about-inflammation/#google_vignette

Gerrard, C. (n.d.). *Celebs with rheumatoid arthritis.* EverydayHealth. https://www.everydayhealth.com/rheumatoid-arthritis/living-with/celebrities-with-rheumatoid-arthritis/

Gunnars, K. (2018, April 23). *Are vegetable and seed oils bad for your health?* Healthline. https://www.healthline.com/nutrition/are-vegetable-and-seed-oils-bad

Herbal Goodness. (2019). *Healthy lifestyle quotes.* Herbalgoodnessco. https://www.herbalgoodnessco.com/

Higuera, V. (2021, November 29). *Whole30: Beginner's guide, what to eat and avoid, and more.* EverydayHealth. https://www.everydayhealth.com/diet-and-nutrition/diet/whole30-program-what-know-before-starting-diet-plan/

Khosla, V. (n.d.). Quotes about Health technology. Quotemaster. https://www.quotemaster.org/health+technology

Lăcătușu, C.-M., Grigorescu, E.-D., Floria, M., Onofriescu, A., & Mihai, B.-M. (2019). The mediterranean diet: From an environment-driven food culture to an emerging medical prescription. *International Journal of Environmental Research and Public Health, 16*(6), 942. https://doi.org/10.3390/ijerph16060942

Liu, W., Li, L., Jiang, J., Wu, M., & Lin, P. (2021). Applications and challenges of cCRISPR-Cas gene-editing to disease treatment in clinics. *Precision Clinical Medicine, 4*(3), 179–191. https://doi.org/10.1093/pcmedi/pbab014

Margaret Rogerson quotes. (n.d.). *Inflammation quotes (8 quotes).* Goodreads. https://www.goodreads.com/quotes/tag/inflammation

Markowiak, P., & Śliżewska, K. (2017). Effects of probiotics, prebiotics, and synbiotics on human health. *Nutrients, 9*(9), 1021. https://doi.org/10.3390/nu9091021

Mikulska, P., Malinowska, M., Ignacyk, M., Szustowski, P., Nowak, J., Pesta, K., Szeląg, M., Szklanny, D., Judasz, E., Kaczmarek, G., Ejiohuo, O. P., Paczkowska-Walendowska, M., Gościniak, A., & Cielecka-Piontek, J. (2023). Ashwagandha (withania somnifera)—current research on the health-promoting activities: A narrative review. *Pharmaceutics, 15*(4), 1057. https://doi.org/10.3390/pharmaceutics15041057

Morey, J. N., Boggero, I. A., Scott, A. B., & Segerstrom, S. C. (2015). Current directions in stress and human immune function. *Current Opinion in Psychology, 5*(1), 13–17. https://doi.org/10.1016/j.copsyc.2015.03.007

Mure, N.S. quotes. (2015, October 15). *EAT! Empower. Adjust. Triumph!: Lose ridiculous weight, succeed on any diet plan, bust through any plateau in 3 empowering steps!* YourSpecs.

Pahwa, R., & Jialal, I. (2019, June 4). Chronic inflammation. *StatPearls Publishing.* https://www.ncbi.nlm.nih.gov/books/NBK493173/

Peng, Y., Ao, M., Dong, B., Jiang, Y., Yu, L., Chen, Z., Hu, C., & Xu, R. (2021). Anti-inflammatory effects of curcumin in the inflammatory diseases: Status, limitations and countermeasures. *Drug Design, Development and Therapy, 15*, 4503–4525. https://doi.org/10.2147/DDDT.S327378

Rafieian-Kopaei, M., Setorki, M., Doudi, M., Baradaran, A., & Nasri, H. (2014). Atherosclerosis: process, indicators, risk factors and new hopes. *International Journal of Preventive Medicine, 5*(8), 927–946. https://www.ncbi.nlm.nih.gov/pmc/articles/PMC4258672/

Ravi, M., Miller, A. H., & Michopoulos, V. (2021). The immunology of stress and the impact of inflammation on the brain and behavior. *BJPsych Advances, 27*(3), 158–165. https://doi.org/10.1192/bja.2020.82

Rediger, J. Quotes. (2020, February 4). Cured: Strengthen Your Immune System and Heal Your Life. Flatiron Books.

Rohn, J. (n.d.).. BrainyQuote. *Jim Rohn quotes.* https://www.brainyquote.com/quotes/jim_rohn_147499

Saini, H. K., Xu, Y.-J., Zhang, M., Liu, P. P., Kirshenbaum, L. A., & Dhalla, N. S. (2005). Role of tumour necrosis factor-alpha and other cytokines in ischemia-reperfusion-induced injury in the heart. *Experimental and Clinical Cardiology, 10*(4), 213–222. https://www.ncbi.nlm.nih.gov/pmc/articles/PMC2716235/

Senthelal, S., & Thomas, M. A. (2018, November 14). Arthritis. *StatPearls Publishing.* https://www.ncbi.nlm.nih.gov/books/NBK518992/

Siddiqui, M. Z. (2011). Boswellia Serrata, a potential antiinflammatory agent: An overview. *Indian Journal of Pharmaceutical Sciences, 73*(3), 255–261.

Sleeydays365. (2023, May 26). *Celebrities who value good quality sleep.* Medium. https://medium.com/@sleepydays365/celebrities-who-value-good-quality-sleep-a94e64deb7a2

Tavakoli, K., Pour-Aboughadareh, A., Kianersi, F., Poczai, P., Etminan, A., & Shooshtari, L. (2021). Applications of CRISPR-Cas9 as an Advanced Genome Editing System in Life Sciences. *BioTech, 10*(3), 14. https://doi.org/10.3390/biotech10030014

Khosla, V.(n.d.). *Quotes about Health technology.* Quotemaster. https://www.quotemaster.org/health+technology

Weil, A. (2006, August 8). *Anti-Inflammatory diet* https://www.drweil.com/diet-nutrition/anti-inflammatory-diet-pyramid/dr-weils-anti-inflammatory-diet/

Widmer, R. J., Flammer, A. J., Lerman, L. O., & Lerman, A. (2015). The mediterranean diet, its components, and cardiovascular disease. *The American Journal of Medicine, 128*(3), 229–238. https://doi.org/10.1016/j.amjmed.2014.10.014

Zamani, M., Mahnaz Rezaei Kelishadi, Damoon Ashtary-Larky, Niusha Amirani, Goudarzi, K., Iman Attackpour Torki, Bagheri, R., Matin Ghanavati, & Omid Asbaghi. (2023, January 10). The effects of green tea supplementation on cardiovascular risk factors: A systematic review and meta-analysis. *Frontlines in Nutrition, 9.* https://doi.org/10.3389/fnut.2022.1084455

Zhang, J.-M., & An, J. (2007). Cytokines, inflammation, and pain. *International Anesthesiology Clinics, 45*(2), 27–37. https://doi.org/10.1097/AIA.0b013e318034194e

Zhu, H. (2014). Acupoints initiate the healing process. *Medical Acupuncture, 26*(5), 264–270. https://doi.org/10.1089/acu.2014.1057